LOVE YOUR DISEASE
Highway to Health

John Harrison, M.D.

PEACOCK BOOKS

Published by
PEACOCK BOOKS
7/22, Ansari Road, Darya Ganj, New Delhi-110002
Phones : +91-11-40775252, 23273880, 23275880, 23280451
Fax : +91-11-23285873
Web : www.atlanticbooks.com
E-mail : orders@atlanticbooks.com

Branch Office
5, Nallathambi Street, Wallajah Road, Chennai-600002
Phones : +91-44-64611085, 32413319
E-mail : chennai@atlanticbooks.com

Peacock Books is an imprint of
Atlantic Publishers and Distributors (P) Ltd.

Printed in India at Nice Printing Press, A-33/3A, Site-IV,
Industrial Area, Sahibabad, Ghaziabad, U.P.

Health in the 3rd Millennium

Thank you to the many people who have made this book possible by their willingness to take the journey of exploration required for healing over the past 35 years since "Love Your Disease It's keeping you healthy" was published.

With courage and insight they've pursued a dream that at times must have appeared beyond their reach.

This book reveals what we all learned.

www.m3health.com

For Tracey Jones,

mother, wife, osteopath

And the children asked that she lay her hands upon them

Acknowledgements

Many thanks to Robyn Harrison and Tim Pulsford who selflessly and tirelessly shaped this work.

Contents

Section 3:
The m3health Program

Introduction

Your doctor can only assist you, not “make you better”.

For healing which is effective and long lasting we need to optimise our own body physiology.

Many treatments are ineffective because our own body physiology is sabotaging them.

This book helps you recover from illness, maintain health and create well-being using the resources provided by the natural course of your life.

One of those resources is your current illness.

There’s nothing to take and no diet, exercise, affirmations, practices, religions or deprivations.

The m3health program heals you by involving you in an exploration of your own life.

It provides a road map to assist you.

Are you ready for such a journey?

Is The m3health Program for Me?

You're the best person to judge what you need and what works for you.

The m3health program is designed to help with any problem, not just health problems. It's effective with psychological problems, relationship impasses, concerns about life direction, childrearing difficulties, work considerations and enjoyment of life issues. It helps you see all these things differently and helps you resolve them.

Over a 45-year period we've been successful in helping people who are familiar with the sort of thoughts and feelings listed in the table on the next two pages.

But is it for me?

Check it out.

Do you recognise yourself?

Is This You?

	YES	NO
There's something wrong with me		
Nothing seems to work		
Why don't these tablets work for me?		
I like to keep up with new developments in health		
I've gone from one doctor to another		
I don't want any more tests		
I've spend a fortune on blood tests, X-Rays, scans etc. and I'm still ill		
If only someone would listen		
I love going to the doctor		
Many people are worse off than me. I shouldn't complain		
There's got to be more to life than this		
I'm never feeling quite right		
There's nothing wrong with me		
If it works I'll give it a go		
I'm so annoyed with having to put up with this		
It scares me		
I've been waiting for something like this to happen		
I feel pretty good, but there's something not quite right		

	YES	NO
I feel tense much of the time		
I guess I'm resigned to a life like this now		
I used to be full of joy and look at me now		
What's the point! I can't be bothered anymore		
I used to be full of life		
No point in getting upset about it		
I've had the wind taken from my sails		
I guess I've never really felt loved		
I'd say that I'm depressed a good part of the time		
I'm OK. They're the problem!		
What's the point in getting angry about it		
I'm always trying to improve my life		
It's so unfair		
The cure is as bad as the condition		
I'm going to really enjoy this program		
I'm OK, but I would like to know more		
I'd like to know how to care for the family better		

If you're familiar with FIVE or so of these questions/ comments then it's likely that the m3health Program could assist you with whatever problems you have in your life right now.

Love Your Disease

The Highway to Health inquiry has developed from the ideas and understandings introduced by the book

Love Your Disease

It's keeping you healthy.(1)

Since the publication of that seminal work over 30 years ago, m3health has been developing and testing a program that will give you direct access to tools for managing your own health and well-being using the principles outlined in "Love your Disease". The program is designed for use in conjunction with other health strategies provided by your doctor and other health attendants.

Over the past thirty years thousands of books about healthcare were written by a multitude of authors, often based upon an idea or hypothesis without regard for clinical experience. Many of the suggested methodologies had little chance of working in the real world. Some treatments that became popular when they showed early promise have proven unsustainable with the passage of time and experience. Highway to Health makes use of those developments shown to be effective in a wide range of people and their problems.

Our approach has now been confirmed by 35 years of clinical experience, and an increasing body of scientific evidence.

The program has been designed so that you can manage the route to recovery yourself, wherever you are and whenever

1. John Harrison, Angus and Robertson (UK and Australia) 1984 and Hay House (USA) 1990.

it suits you. It provides a framework that prompts readers to move forward at a pace that suits them.

You're guided through a process that maximises your own body's healing mechanisms. The program provides material to which you respond and then it uses those responses to optimise your own healing. The three major responses that the Program draws upon are your thoughts, feelings and actions. It makes use of the actual problem to solve itself and draws upon nature in innovative ways.

Highway to Health is the book form of the m3health Program, the recovery and prevention program contained in the website, Health in the 3rd Millennium, found at www.m3health.com

The m3health program is exciting, and fun to undertake.

It turns upside down many of our notions of cause and cure.

You can use the program again if a subsequent need arises.

Its revelations continue for life.

IS THIS PROGRAM FOR YOU?

Have you tried the questions in the chapter "Is the m3health program for me?"

Our journey begins with an overview of some fundamental concepts.

A description of the Program topics appears on page 15.

But before we get into the m3health Program proper, let's take a look at some usual comments people tend to make about doctors and health. Are you, or is someone you know, in these pages?

"WHAT...! NOT MORE TABLETS!"

"I'm taking so many pills I rattle when I walk!"

"They used to help but they don't any longer."

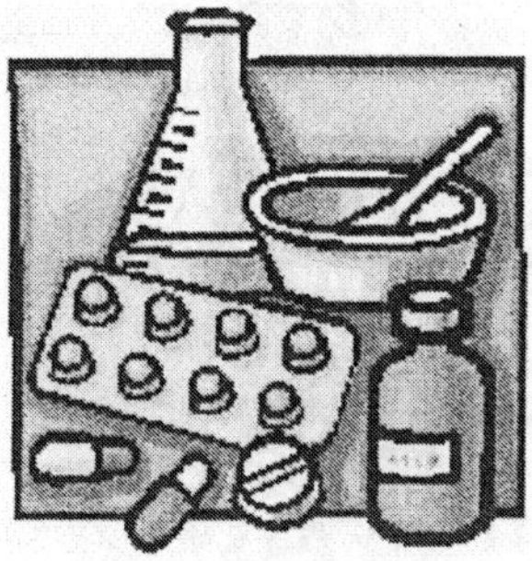

"There's always a new pill which is supposed to work better and have fewer side effects than the last!"

"I need to start helping my doctor rather than insisting he give me all these pills."

Why does a tablet, pill, potion, pharmaceutical or drug work with one person and not another?

Why did they work before and not now?

Is there something about me which is different?

Can I do something about it?

Can I reduce my dependence on tablets?

"WHAT...! NOT MORE TESTS!"

"I've had every test imaginable and still no diagnosis!"

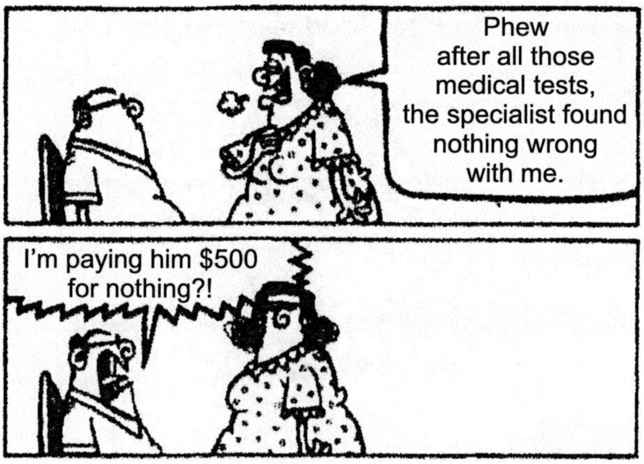
Phew
after all those
medical tests,
the specialist found
nothing wrong
with me.
I'm paying him $500
for nothing?!

© Chew Chew Straits Times Jan. 14 2001

"I've spent a fortune on blood tests, X-rays, scans, etc. and I'm still ill."

"There's got to be something which I can do to help."

"I've had so much blood taken it's a wonder I'm still alive."

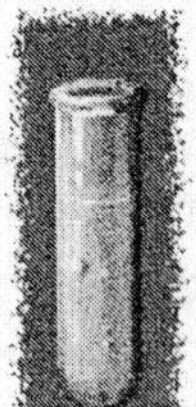

Medical investigations have made spectacular contributions to medical science in recent years and have saved multiple lives.

For serious illness, investigations need to be thorough and exhaustive, and sometimes attending different doctors is necessary before a test proves vital in establishing a diagnosis which leads to successful therapy.

However, more tests do not necessarily mean a greater chance of finding a remedy.

Complex, expensive tests carried out in hospitals or clinics are not without their own risks.

We cannot rely totally upon our doctor and her investigations. There's a part we need to play as well.

How do you know how many tests to have?

"I'M UNDER THE DOCTOR"

"My doctor's great, but I'm just not getting better!"

"She's tried to talk to me about my involvement in my own recovery but I haven't wanted to listen."

"We need to talk but we're both too busy!"

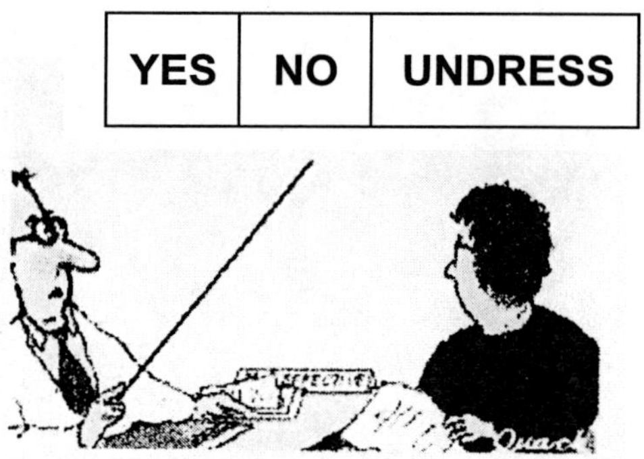

©Quack MD

"My doctor's really done everything he could."

"My doctor said that I was very lucky. She got the problem just in time—but it keeps on coming back."

"I've gone from one doctor to another."

"My doctor's been very straight with me. He says he's done all he can."

"I don't want her to refer me for more tests or to another specialist."

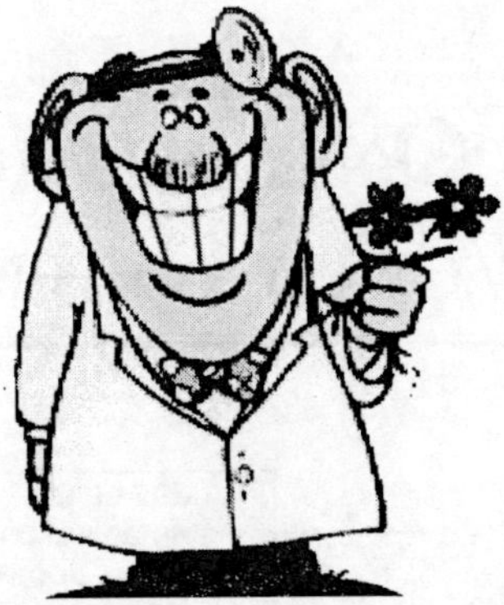

Your doctor has more knowledge about medicine than you, but you know a lot more about you than he does, and probably a lot more about this disease than you both realise.

What can you do to start getting better, rather than relying totally on him?

Recovery needs to be a partnership.

"If Only Someone Would Listen"

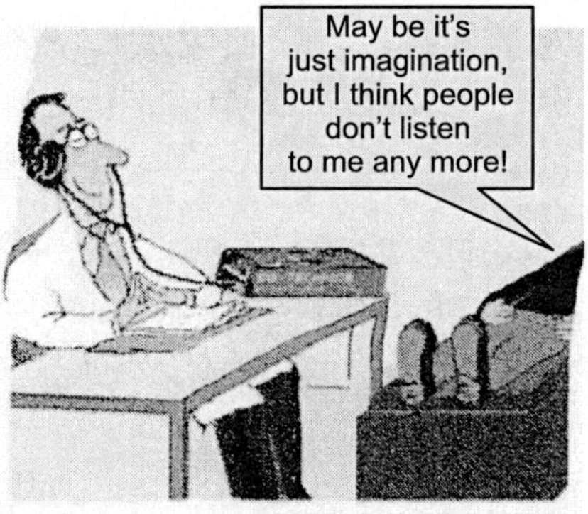
May be it's
just imagination,
but I think people
don't listen
to me any more!

©Quack MD

"My doctor's very kind but he doesn't have the time to listen."

The art of listening is time consuming and hard to build into a busy practice.

Our doctor does the best she can with the restraints upon her, but we must also make the time to listen to ourselves and try and find a role we can play in our own recovery.

The m3health Program provides an opportunity to find that role and play that part.

Our Contribution to Wellness

Two parties are involved in your recovery from illness.

One is your health advisor.

The other is you.

This book is for you.

M3health helps you fulfil your contribution to your own health.

The m3health Program is a new route to wellness. Developed by health practitioners over forty years, it's now available in this book and on the Internet at www.m3health.com

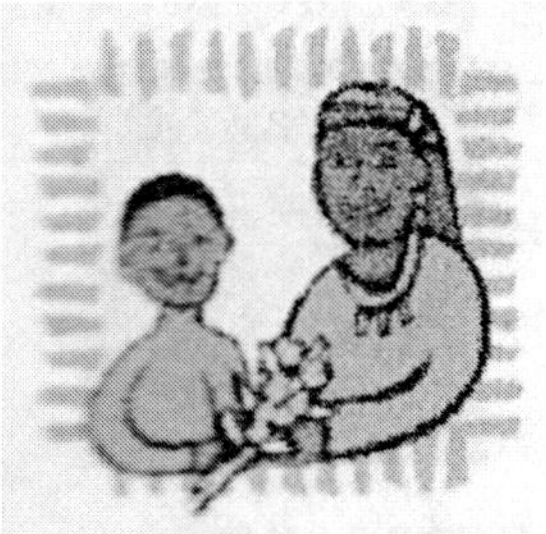

Your own doctor may not have had the opportunity of discussing with you how you can best work together to solve your problem.

The Program can be used in conjunction with all therapies whilst attending any health practitioner. It evokes the healing potential within the patient himself, and is designed for all health and personal problems. It assists both cure and prevention. The program helps us to see our condition differently, and in doing so frees up healing. The program is exciting to undertake and its revelations continue for life.

It helps you benefit from the services of health practitioners and the investigations and the treatments which those clinicians recommend.

Each of us must take responsibility for carefully assessing all medical treatment which we elect to undertake. Fortunately, a broad spectrum of opinions from a wide range of health disciplines is available to assist you.

> ***A cornerstone of m3health's philosophy is that we all do the very best we can in the circumstances........always***

M3health's view is that as biological organisms, we cannot do something which is not in our interests, much as we protest otherwise in the hope of maintaining the self-critical belief that "There's something wrong with me!"

Our thoughts, feelings, actions, beliefs and attitudes may be making us ill and preventing our recovery. Are you ready to explore this?

The m3health Program is ready to help you.

Summary of m3health Program Chapters

1. First Step	A thorough evaluation of your current therapy.
2. Your Family	Beliefs and attitudes acquired within the family may be inhibiting our healing potential.
3. Illness confirms beliefs	We say "Life sucks!" because we're ill. However, we may be ill because we already believe "Life sucks!"
4. Who am I?	What has our personality got to do with our illness and our recovery from it?
5. Responses to being ill	Illness is emotive. It provides a powerful opportunity to unmask thoughts and feelings that have remained hidden for a long time and may be keeping you ill.
6. Glossary of Terms	The origin of terms such as "dis-ease", "re-present", "respons-ibility" are discussed and the contribution an understanding of them makes to both the origins of, and the recovery from, illness.
7. Knowledge	How what you "know" may be stopping you from recovering. Read the last sentence again. Did you understand it the first time?

8. First nature and second nature	We're all familiar with the term "second nature" without ever considering that it implies the existence of "first nature". What is first nature and how can we involve it in our own healing?
9. The immune system	How our thoughts and feelings limit our natural responses.
10. Thoughts	One of the most powerful causes of pain and suffering comes from our thoughts. We need to use this powerful force, but not by trying to change what we think, and certainly not by replacing "negative" thoughts with "positive" thoughts, but by allowing all thoughts to visit us.......and to leave us. Stop thinking and allow yourself to be "thunk".
11. Feelings	The four basic emotions of anger, sadness, fear and joy and their integral relationship to the proper functioning of our immune and endocrine (hormonal) systems.
12. Express or Repress	The effect on our health of repressing emotions and what happens when we take the risk of expressing them.
13. Anger	Does it deserve its bad press? What's the difference between anger and violence? Can we use healthy anger to assist healing?
14. Practising Feeling Emotions	Unlocking feelings to unlock the immune and endocrine systems.
15. Fear	At the bottom of many an illness. Anxiety and panic unmasked.

16. Sadness	Usually more of a problem with men. It's important to involve the full range of physiological responses, such as crying, in an m3health Program of recovery.
17. Joy	Putting joy back into life with laughter and love.
18. The Feral Healer	Unleashing an old friend to help you.
19. Half-way review	A review of the journey thus far.
20. Moving Right Along	Taking your time.
21. Doing	The obsession with "doing" may be restricting your healing.
22. Et tu Bruté?	Are we are our worst enemy when it comes to getting better?
23. Cause and Cure	The forgotten origins of illness and the ignored main healing element.
24. Self Acceptance	Why we criticise ourselves and how we might use that realisation to move on.
25. Judgement	The decommissioning of the prime mover of chronic dis-ease.
26. Being	Most of us have forgotten how to "be". Being isn't lost, only hidden. We may need to re-experience it to heal ourselves.
27. Self	At the core of our healing nature or first nature lies an untapped resource.
28. Meditation	Practising doing *nothing* so that your body can achieve *something*.

29. Finding our Selfs — Hiding under the canopy of our defences is something we mislaid, rather than lost. We "find ourselves" doing, thinking and feeling.....something.....it doesn't matter much what. Find your "self" and healing won't be far behind.

30. Acceptance — Accepting ourselves, whoever, whenever, however, wherever we are. What does this involve? Is it something that you "**Do**"?

31. Letting Go — Not something that you *do*, but something that shows up.

32. Control — *"You're out of control"* becomes music to your ears when you realise the cost of staying *"In control"*.

33. Guilt, Fault and Blame — These powerful emotions often contribute to illness and must be harnessed for healing.

34. Should and Ought — Remember these. How do we know what's best for us? Perhaps we don't. Then how do we know what we "should" be doing or what we "ought" to have done?

Section 1: Fundamentals

The Journey Begins

1
A HEALING LIFE

The only thing that can truly heal us is our own life

Life heals us, if we let it
It makes us happy, if we honour it
It loves us, if we're open to it
It excites us, if we're up for it
Life heals us, when we let it

This book shows you how to heal yourself using your own life circumstances.

A Journey, a personal Program or an Inquiry often starts when we find that there's something wrong with us, or we have some problem that won't go away. The m3health program takes respondents through an exciting and gentle journey of rediscovering their own lives and resuming their place in them.

The resources we require already surround us.

Healing happens when we stop trying to heal ourselves and allow nature to heal us, a job for which 15 million years of evolution has equipped it.

Life heals us when we let it.

2

Maximising Our Immune and Endocrine Systems

The m3health program improves the functioning of the immune and endocrine systems of the body. These two systems are vital for maintaining health and recovering from illness.

If these systems are not working properly, no treatment, whatever it is, will be effective.

The **immune system** maintains our body's healthy relationship with external elements such as bacteria, viruses, allergens and pollutants. Living organisms are a vital component of our internal and external health environment. Our health is integrated with organisms primarily within our gut and on our skin. Should an imbalance occur between us and our environmental co-inhabitants, the immune system attempts to restore the balance.

The **endocrine system** is responsible for the internal functioning of the organs. If an imbalance occurs within the body the endocrine system corrects it.

The m3health program identifies and rectifies restrictions upon these two systems, making them more responsive.

Such restrictions take the form of left over attitudes, beliefs, opinions and emotions that we've acquired during our lives. They're the defence or protective mechanisms that we've assembled in order to feel safe. But sometimes they obstruct our otherwise healthy relationships with other living organisms, and obstruct healing. Many of them are well past their "use by" date.

The m3health program releases them and in so doing frees the mind and subsequently the body physiology to heal us.

The m3health program facilitates healing. At the end of the Program, you probably won't be able to say how you became well.

3
Being Available

"If you're very, very careful, then nothing bad, or good, will ever happen to you".

Ashleigh Brilliant

Being available means being open to new understandings. It means taking a risk.

The risk is not to life or limb usually, but to old opinions and views which, whilst they've kept us safe until now, may well be getting in our way of taking the next step in our life, like recovery from this illness, or preventing the next.

Being available means that you don't know the answers before you begin.

> ***"If, just if...there's something in this new way of looking at health, I'll be well placed to benefit from it. I'm not sure how it works but I'll give it a try".***

Being un-available means that we're sure..., certain..., right..., positive that we know. Nothing new can penetrate our consciousness. We have fixed ideas about how something will look if it's going to work. This guarantees that any new advance in healing will pass us by. When we dismiss something out of the ordinary as just so much mumbo jumbo, as unscientific, unproven, anecdotal....we fail to acknowledge that this is our fear speaking, not the objective analysis we claim it to be.

The addiction to what we "know" is a very seductive addiction, and one of the most difficult to overcome. It's most persistent form is seen in the addiction to being "right".

When it comes to healing, no two people are equally available.

WHAT'S YOUR POTENTIAL?

Becoming available isn't easy. We'll fool ourself that we're available but we won't be. We'll claim that we're ready to see life with new eyes. But our old conditioning and our old defences will fight to interpret new discoveries in terms that will keep us feeling comfortable, urging us to return to the safety of the known.

Opening our mind is not enough. We must open our senses, our heart, our soul....our everything.

This lifetime journey of discovery is the same for all of us. You, me and all our fellow human beings, doctors and doormen, patients and poets, builders and ballerinas alike.

4

Health Partnerships – The New Deal

Nobody else, however qualified, skilled and well-intentioned, can "make us better."

They can help, but in the end it's up to us. We need a more active role in our own healing rather than being passive recipients of health care. We need to be in **partnership** with our health practitioner.

A new **Health Contract** between us and our practitioner gives us a new active role and new responsibilities.

This book provides the tools to enable patients to fulfil their new role within such a Health Contract, even if the contract is not explicitly negotiated. That role is to create a "fertile environment" in which our physician's treatment can work most effectively. This is our side of the new **Health Partnership** bargain.

Playing an enhanced role in our own health does not remove the need for a medical attendant. The doctor's role in the Health Partnership is essential, but different from ours. The selection of doctors and their treatments is as important as ever, and the m3health program helps us to make those choices.

Long-term health comes from helping our doctor help us, and from helping ourselves.

5
HELPING YOUR DOCTOR

Your doctor has more knowledge about medicine than you, but you know a lot more about you than he does and probably a lot more about this disease than you both realise.

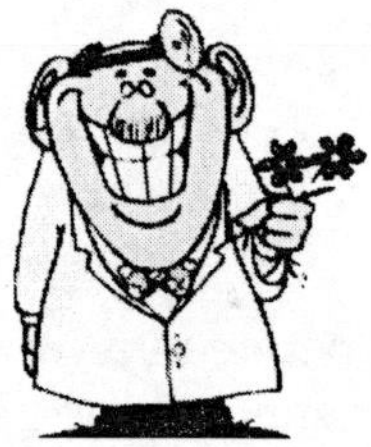

(our doctor again)

There are Providers of healthcare (doctors, hospitals etc.) and there are Consumers of healthcare (patients).

Good health depends primarily upon the consumer, not the provider of health services.

The lack of preparation of the patient is the major reason why many treatments either fail, or make the patient worse. Doctor induced disease (iatrogenic disease) is currently believed to be the fourth highest cause of death in the United States.

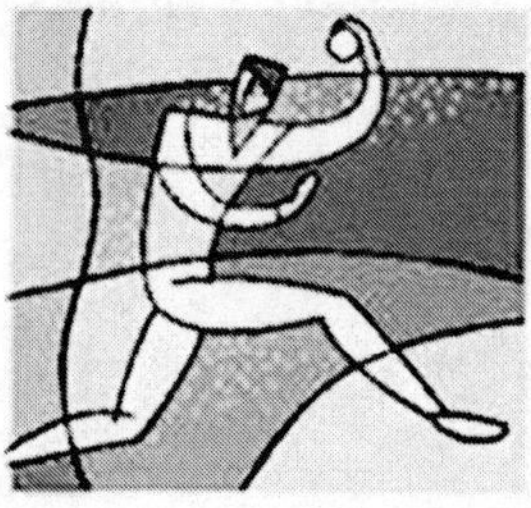

Whilst medical science and medical practice has become very focused upon technology and medications, the patient side of the healing equation is just as important.

Lifestyle, diet, exercise, Return to Work and relaxation are now part of the doctor's prescription. However, these account for only a small portion of the patient's potential contribution to their own health.

The principle factors behind many of the illnesses presenting every day to general practitioners across the world are psycho-social.

Attitudes, beliefs, opinions and emotions related to jobs, work colleagues, finances, education, health matters, relationships, raising families and everyday living create stressors. These stressors are at the bottom of many illnesses, and failure to address them results in failure to recover, and in chronic disease, whatever the treatment. These are the areas that can be addressed by the patient and as such they constitute the patient portion of the health contract.

Few people, consumers and suppliers of healthcare alike, have been prepared to address this obvious fact, because neither believed it was in their interests to do so. The doctor has wanted to remain in control of healthcare delivery and the patient has wanted to hand responsibility for his health to somebody else.

HOW HAS THIS CHANGED?

The public has become more informed. There's an increased understanding that "dispensed health" is not entirely safe. Much medical research, particularly in the field of pharmacology, is less objective than might be expected.

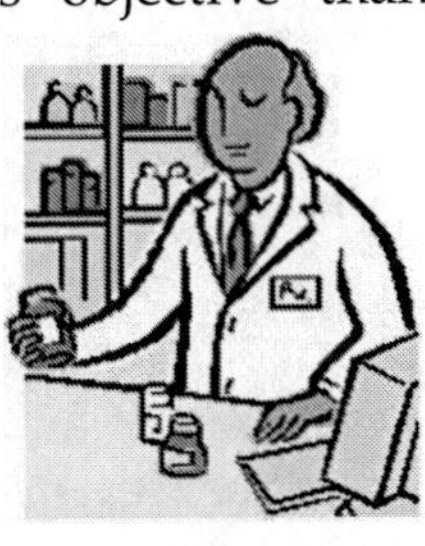

Recent revelations indicate that neither prescribers (doctors) nor consumers (patients) can rely upon information supplied by drug manufacturers. In addition drug resistant organisms have developed in response to overuse of antibiotics, making hospitals dangerous places to be. Iatrogenic (doctor induced) illness is now the fourth highest killer in the United States. These, and other health matters, are now publicly known.

"Perhaps one-third of all medical spending – some $800 billion dollars – may be unnecessary, out-of-date, or even dangerous treatments."

Business Week August 26, 2002

"Close to a trillion dollars spent on healthcare is unnecessary."

"Reducing Waste in Healthcare." *Health Affairs* 2012

The fact that 70% of Americans explore their condition on the Net as well as consulting a health professional, demonstrates that people are now doing their own research and taking a greater interest in their own health. They're preparing themselves to take on a new role.

The advent of PROMs (Patient Reported Outcome Measures) provides a direct report of medical interventions, by patients. For the past 100 years, doctors have been judging the effectiveness of their treatment of patients, now it's the turn of the patients.

We can increase the effectiveness of recovery from and prevention of illness, but we must play an increasing role in managing the process. People must recognise that in seeking medical help they are effectively entering into a partnership with their medical attendant. If the partnership is to work well they must take responsibility for the patient component, and not expect all of the effort to come from the other party.

We can no longer expect anyone else to "make us better".

That's great, but what's available to assist those people wanting to play a more active role in their own health?

Alternative or complementary medicine consumer products such as herbs, exercise products, applications etc. are products in which the consumer is, once again, asked to rely upon the expertise of someone else. And once again many will be disappointed. The products will not work any better than orthodox drugs (mostly they're less effective but with fewer side effects), because the ground in which they're expected to work is not prepared, i.e. the patient is not fertile ground for healing. There's virtually nothing available to help the patient help himself, without recourse to health products or health provider services.

The m3health program assists people maximise their own healing potential.

It does this by addressing the underlying factors affecting health. Old attitudes, beliefs and opinions as well as left over unresolved emotions cause or contribute to illness, both physical and psychological. The m3health program prepares the patient to respond beneficially to medical treatment by identifying and removing obstacles to healing. These obstacles restrict the ability of the immune and the endocrine systems to respond to immediate threats. In the longer term, systems which are prevented from effectively protecting us, are redirected to attack us.

M3health has addressed these issues for over 40 years of clinical practice and has developed a program that the patient undertakes himself, with the assistance of his practitioner, should both parties desire it.

Whilst the patient is attending a practitioner of his or her own choosing, the m3health program works to clear any obstacles which may be stopping the treatment being successful.

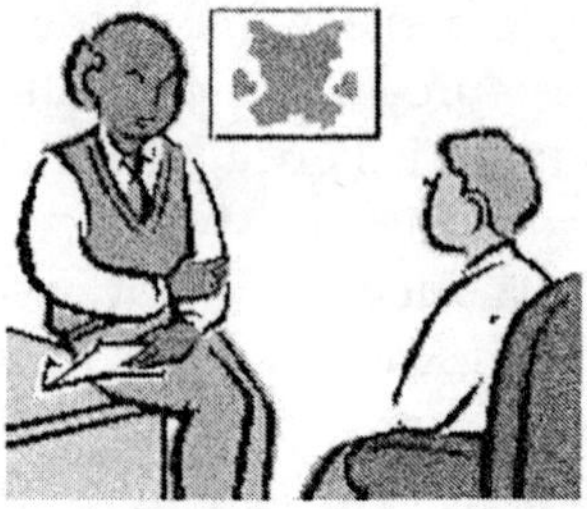

Health is the most researched subject on the internet and more books are sold on health than any other topic.

Conventional medical treatments have a major place in health but are not as effective without the patient's contribution to healing.

Complementary treatments are also augmented by the patient's involvement in his own treatment.

The cost of all medical practice is reduced when the patient becomes an active participant in treatment.

The challenge for health in the third millennium is to create a "fertile patient environment".

Section 2: Getting Prepared

Healing Panoramas

1
Go For It

You know, sometimes we just have to do something different if we want to solve a problem, especially if it's been hanging around for too long.

Sometimes we just have to say:

"Enough is enough. I've given that treatment a good run and I still have the problem, so what can I do differently?"

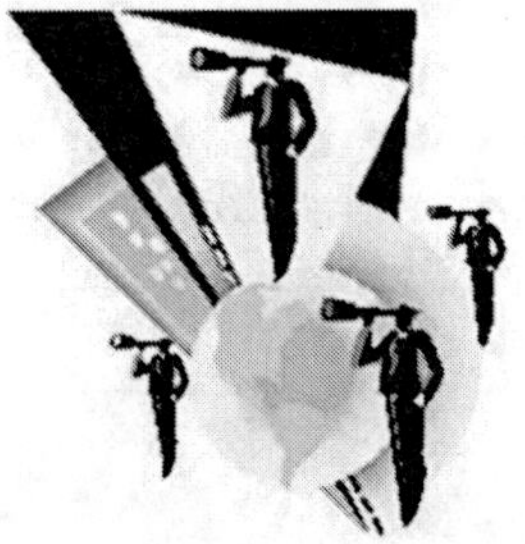

We might need to approach our doctor and say to him that we feel the need to try something different. He or she will be available to help as much as possible, but for this part of your own cure you might need to take charge of your own exploration. Your doctor may have taken the conventional route as far as he's able at this point in time, and may be happy to assist you to help yourself.

We can also help you. The m3health Program is carefully designed to help those people who've arrived at the realisation that now is the time to become more involved in their own health. The section "Going Further" in this book and the *subscription information* page on *www.m3health.com* gives comprehensive information about additional services that m3health provides.

Now is an exciting time. It's like the first page in a book of blank pages, inviting you to write a new approach to you, your health, your life. It invites you to take a chance and step into a new scenario, to embark upon a journey of discovering what you can personally do to recover from this illness and avoid another. When you're ready, we're ready.

The Program chapters provide a detailed investigation into the thoughts and emotions behind continuing ill health, and provide multiple perspectives to assist you move beyond your current situation and into wellness. They're designed for all physical and psychological diseases, as well as personal, relationship, emotional, sexual and work related problems. Indeed they're designed to give you a new insight into all suffering.

The **m3** health series is meant to be your lifelong health companion. Not only your health companion, but a guide to stimulate and encourage you to follow your own unique journey. We hold your hand in the early days and provide a range of signposts and checkpoints. Then, before you know it, whoosh, you're off and flying.

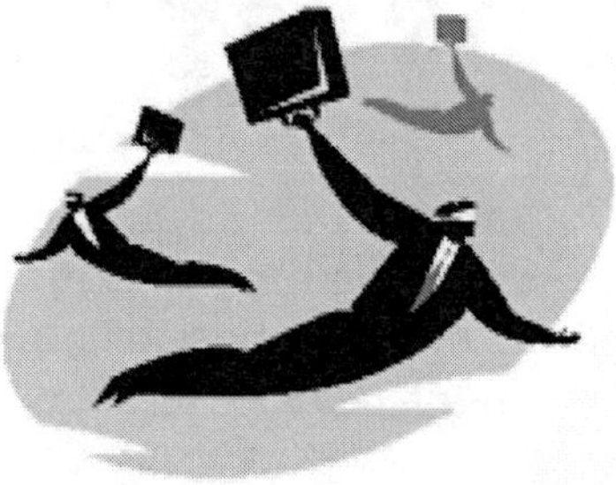

You'll come to realise the cost of total reliance on others and their expertise, for whilst they may remove symptoms that we didn't like, another problem may arise in the place of the one just removed, or is caused by the treatment of the first problem. In order to continuously heal we must address the very nature of illness and health. We need to do this ourselves, with our doctor's help.

The m3health Program is energising, enlightening, revealing and very, very forgiving.

Many have told us that they've revisited the program years after their initial involvement and have been taken to a new level of understanding.

It opens up new ways of viewing many of life's difficulties.

We invite you to take this journey with us.

2
Getting Out of Our Own Way (so that healing can happen)

Are you in the way of your own healing?

What can you do to assist your own healing process?

Are you fertile ground for healing?

Are you allowing healing to happen?

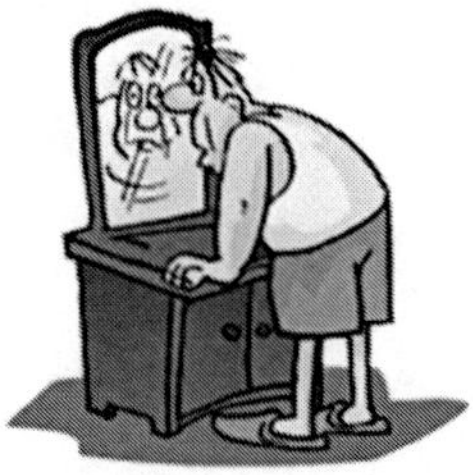

Are you obstructing healing by trying to force it?

Are you expecting your doctor to take total responsibility for you?

This book provides you with the opportunity of contributing to your own recovery and long-term health.

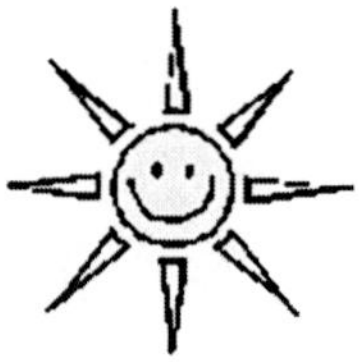

All therapies — from drugs to massage, from surgery to homoeopathy have the potential to "work" — providing we get out of the way and let them.

We can either obstruct therapy (usually without realising it) or we can assist and amplify its effect.

3
HEALTH PARTNERSHIP

Health is a complex matter and some of the elements that contribute to health are less obvious than others.

Common sense dictates that we use what works.

In this era of spectacular pharmaceutical medicine, laser surgery and gene therapy it's easy to overlook one of the most potent factors in health and recovery. That element is the patient himself.

Whilst modern medicine has become very adept at categorising a disease and treating the symptoms of that disease with drugs and other means, the person with the disease is still a source of healing in his own right.

Some conditions may require the patient's involvement if a longer term cure is to be achieved.

Failure to get better is one indicator that the patient himself may be standing in the way of recovery – but what to do about it?

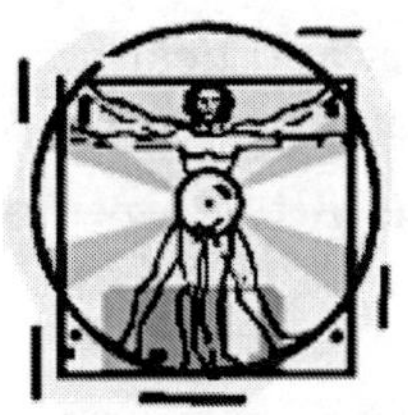

This book is for those people who believe that alongside the doctor and modern medicine, and in conjunction with any alternative or complementary health treatments, there's an element to health and well-being which is most effectively addressed by the sufferer himself.

It doesn't diminish the role of any practitioner, orthodox or otherwise, nor promotes nor discredits any type of treatment. Rather it aims to maximise all therapies by involving the patient in that element of his own recovery and ongoing health to which he can contribute.

The patient establishes a "health partnership" with his medical attendant in which the patient is the chief stakeholder.

Much is unknown about why some of us get ill and fail to recover, while others recover quickly or rarely become ill at all. Although the latest advances in modern medicine have enriched the lives of many people, the human being behind the condition will always be a rewarding area of inquiry and the focus of the m3health Program.

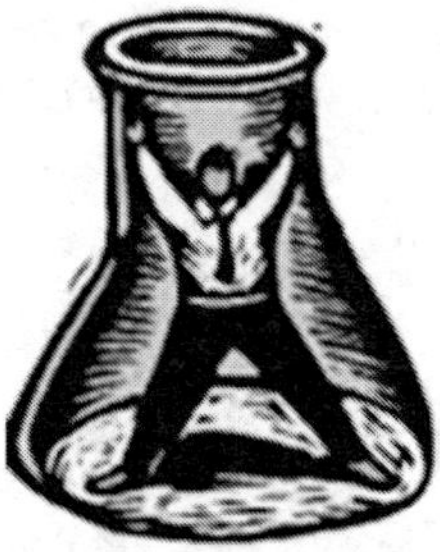

Medical science, doctors and health practitioners facilitate one component of your health journey.

But the vehicle and the driver on the Highway to Health, is you.

4

To Suffer or Not to Suffer

Suffering can be used to discover what lies beneath the symptoms of disease...helping in our quest for recovery and prevention.

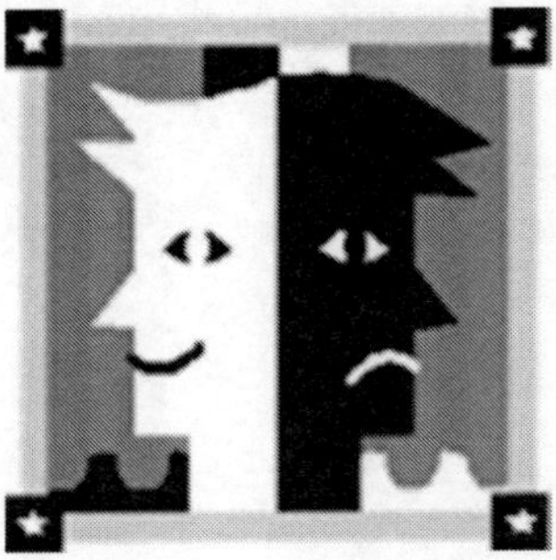

Suffering usually involves uncomfortable thoughts, feelings, and sensations. We need to use these, not just get rid of them using drugs, painkillers and the like. This is akin to throwing the baby out with the bathwater.

If we eliminate our suffering but learn nothing from it then the suffering may return...this time stronger than before.

On the other hand, if a disease is self limiting, easily managed and disappears without consequence or recurrence, there's no need to do anything other than relieve the symptoms and end the suffering.

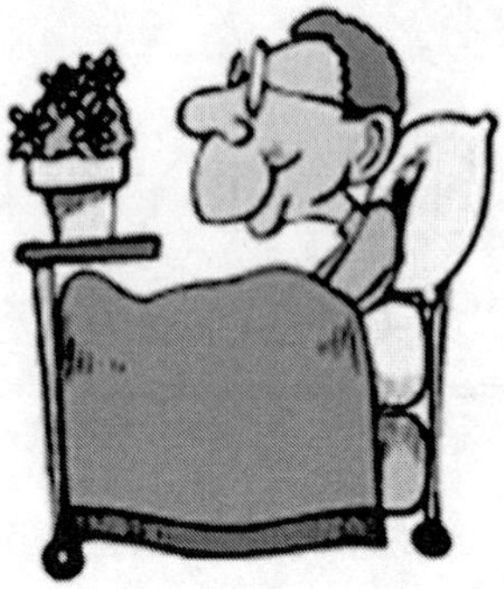

The severity of the disease and whether it recurs usually dictates which course to take. If it keeps on coming back, we may benefit from taking a look at what's behind it.

5
Is There an Obstruction to Healing?

Whether or not healing is being prevented from taking its natural course is subjective. Sometimes you might feel that the condition is hanging on for too long although you're being advised that the timeframe is not unusual. At other times both you and your medical advisor may agree that you should be better by now.

Below are a few questions which you might ask yourself in order to determine if you've really recovered or if you've perhaps come to accept chronic ill health, forgetting what it was like to be really well.

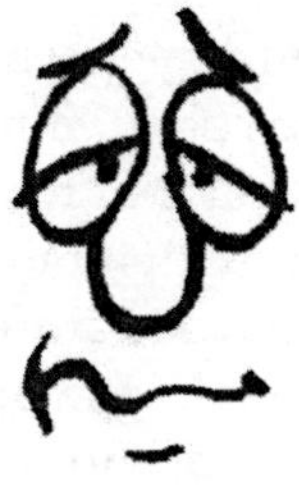

In responding to these questions, it helps to have an initial response that you don't edit. Just let whatever comes up, come up. Later you may have another response. As there are no right and wrong answers, what matters is that you have a response consisting of thoughts, emotions, perhaps bodily sensations and maybe even do something. No-one else is commenting on your responses, so you may want to review them yourself later. For this reason it helps to tape them or write them down. We also offer the option of an electronic log and a self assessment tool, m3checkit on www.m3health.com.

If no-one else is commenting upon them, how do your responses help you?

By witnessing your own responses, listening to them with new ears, seeing them with new eyes, feeling them with expanded emotions, your relationship with your responses changes. You now see the problem to which you were responding, differently.

It no longer has the hold on you it had, for it wasn't really the problem.

Your response to the matter was the real problem. As you free yourself from your controlled responses, your immune system likewise frees itself.

Chronic disease is characterised by an under-functioning immune system. The m3health Program is designed to free up the immune system and remove the disease.

If we respond to another person, doctor, psychiatrist, healer or guru, we focus much of our energy upon being judged by that person. We cast her in the role of a parent, often a benevolent parent we never had, hoping that finally we'll be approved of. By so doing we become more defended, not less defended, and our immune system continues to suffer. We may have replaced the criticism of ourselves with the approval of someone else, but this matters little to an immune system labouring under the weight of any judgements, no matter whether "good" or "bad".

By considering our own responses we become our own parent, judging ourselves less and enjoying ourselves more.

The process of inquiring augments or enhances the body's own healing mechanisms. During the m3health Program inquiry into you and your life, the thoughts, feelings and actions that arise in the course of the inquiry assist healing. Concluding, deciding and judging are less helpful.

"Hullo Mr Respondent, Dr Mirror will see you now."

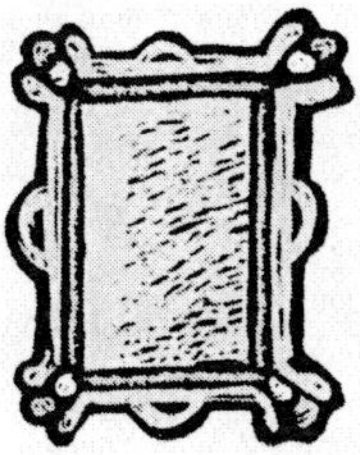

- Are you suffering from any complaint at the moment?
- How long have you had it?
- Was it diagnosed?
- Did you have any investigations?
- Were you referred to a specialist?
- Were you hospitalised?
- Did you receive a course of treatment?
- Was your course of recovery uneventful?
- Did you recover within the timeframe your medical advisor suggested you would?
- Did you take any medication?
- Did you get a second opinion?
- Did you either feel inclined or did you actually attend a practitioner of a discipline different from your original doctor, e.g. an "alternative" or "complementary" medical practitioner?
- Have you had this condition previously?
- Was your recovery easier on the previous occasion?
- Are you unhappy with the medical advice or treatment that you've received for this complaint?
- Do you have feelings of being ignored or dis-respected by the doctor/s?
- Are you of the belief that this problem is likely to return?
- Do you believe that you can improve your state of health?

- Are you willing to accept your current level of well-being?
- Has there been a suggestion that this condition has a "psychological" basis?
- What was your response to that suggestion?
- Do you want to become more active in your own recovery?
- Are you willing to help your doctor to get you better?
- Is all of this pissing you right off?

All your responses (thoughts, feelings, actions) are significant. Some you'll like and others you won't. Some you'll think are right and others wrong, some appropriate and others not. All are to be allowed and eventually welcomed if healing is to happen.

No response needs editing. Mostly we don't have a clue what the response is about or where it came from. "Knowing" these things tends to slow healing, not facilitate it.

Being prepared to accept any response, thought, feeling or action, wherever it comes from, is to remain within the inquiry and not close off the process.

We've been taught that knowing and certainty are good and that uncertainty and irresolution are bad. Staying open is often annoying and can bring uncomfortable feelings to the surface. These will pass.

Come back to the process later if you're feeling too irritated to continue.

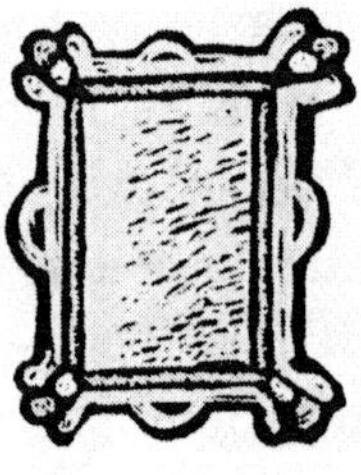

6
COMPROMISED HEALING

- If our disease is one from which other people seem to recover and we don't, we may be stopping ourselves from getting better.
- If nobody is able to recover from a particular disease then presumably that disease is too powerful for any human healing mechanisms.
- If a few people defeat the disease perhaps their immune systems are operating more efficiently than ours. Why?

What might compromise our own healing capabilities?

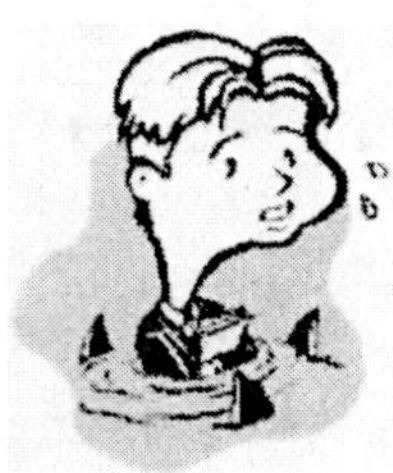

The body is always trying to cure itself of both physical and psychological imbalances. This natural "homeostasis" has guaranteed the survival and evolution of the human species.

The biological mechanisms for achieving this are complex. They're already built into the human organism — we don't have to *know* how they work nor make them work. However, we might have to learn how to stop hindering them.

Consider the simple example of a splinter that has gone deeply into our foot. The body pushes the splinter to the surface, usually with some inflammation, and then expels it. It does this because we're healthier when we're free of the splinter, and our biology is programmed to have us be as healthy as possible. The splinter may have been there for a long time.

In the case of a psychological problem, the same need of the human organism to be as healthy as possible initiates processes that try and resolve the problem. We will be directed, often out of our awareness, towards a set of circumstances that may assist us in expelling the "psychological splinter".

When we place ourselves in a situation that could help us to sort out an unresolved issue, that situation is "representing" the issue.

It's very important that we understand what "represent" means, otherwise we try and change uncomfortable situations without making good use of their healing potential.

"Re-present" means presenting again, bringing the incomplete matter up again. Pronounced with the "present" component of re-present to sound like "present" as in present time, re-"present" means that the old issue resurfaces in the present time in order to be dealt with, i.e. it is....re-"present"-ed.

Physical and psychological diseases or discomforts try and work themselves out of the body and mind in order for us to be as healthy as possible. If we aren't as healthy as we could be, this process is probably being interrupted or curtailed. In order to recover, we consciously and subconsciously go searching for situations in which the underlying matters can be resolved further.

To resolve a recurring or lingering illness we might benefit from investigating what past events it may be representing or re-"present"-ing.

This is an Inquiry. There are no "answers" from the m3health Program. It's ongoing, and it allows for new perspectives and realisations as we proceed.

It's never complete.

If there are matters in our past causing us irritation, they may be trying to work themselves to the surface so as to be completed. The current illness is one way of doing that, bringing into the present something from the past that's unfinished – a "psychological splinter".

If a disease is easily managed by our immune system and is cured, then there's no underlying need demanding re-"present"-ation. It will not be "re-present-ed" because it's already finished or past. If the underlying issue is not completed, then the current illness provides a contemporary vehicle capable of being used to further resolve the issue. This is pro-survival.

During the m3health program we'll explore in great depth how an illness that's representing itself is fulfilling two imperatives.

- The first is to reaffirm the opinions and beliefs of the sufferer that lead to the illness in the first place, e.g. "I'm a hopeless case. There's nothing I can do."
- The second is to provide a set of circumstances in which to resolve the disease, e.g. "There's got to be something behind me suffering for all this time."

The m3health Program provides a framework in which the "psychological splinter" can work itself to the surface and be expelled.

Illness that represents an underlying problem is not going to be cured whilst the underlying matter remains unfinished. The issue keeps seeking out situations in which to place the human organism so that renewed efforts are made to resolve it.

Physical complaints bring up psychological issues, such as left over sadness, for example—and psychological complaints nearly always have physical symptoms attached.

An old emotional or psychological problem may be represented by a new physical or emotional "re-presentation" of itself. There's no rigid boundary between the physical and the psychological, and physiologists acknowledge that they're interdependent – or different representations of the same thing.

If you have a physical problem which won't go away it may well be related to a psychological problem which hasn't gone away either.

7
THE INQUIRY PROCESS

The m3health program is an inquiry.

What are the characteristics of an Inquiry?

To inquire is to look with new eyes and not with one's mind already made up about "how things are". In an Inquiry, certainty is replaced by uncertainty. Uncertainty acknowledges that healing may lie beyond "knowing".

- The m3health Program is open-ended, which means that it doesn't aim for a conclusion.
- It admits any realisation, recognition or information even though they may not conform with accepted knowledge or known "facts".
- It requires the inquirer to be prepared to experience some discomfort or fear in entering into areas previously avoided.
- It assumes that there are no experts and avoids seeking the "truth", preferring to recognise the subjectivity of views and "facts" in the personal field.
- Its relevance is limited.

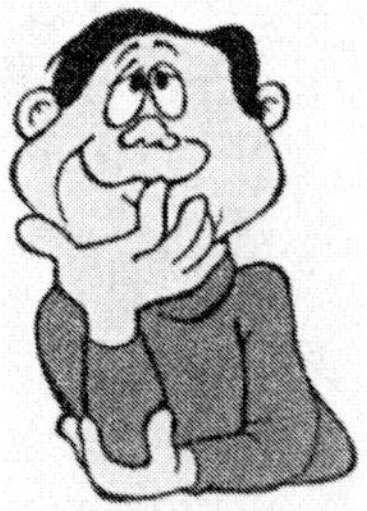

- It recognises that "right" and "wrong" interpretations are unhelpful.
- It does not require that "progress" is made.
- It has no timeframe to which it must adhere.
- An Inquiry is not dependent upon conventional wisdom nor upon scientific theses.
- An Inquiry is free to explore areas which have no obvious connection with the m3health Program.
- It does not seek to validate or to justify itself.
- An Inquiry has no intention.

How can the m3health Inquiry help me?

The m3health program releases your healing potential.

How does that work?

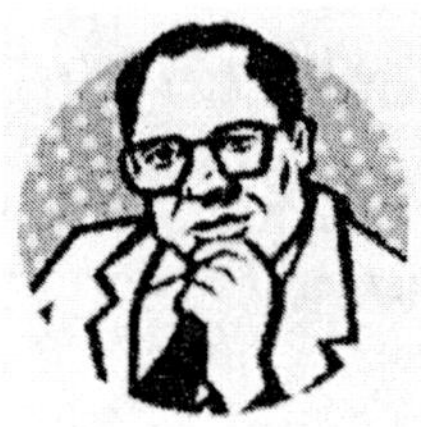

The body has evolved powerful, complex healing mechanisms over millions of years. Two systems vitally concerned with maintaining health are the **immune** system and the **endocrine** system. The former keeps us in a healthy co-existence with our environment, while the latter maintains the internal equilibrium. This latter function is called homoeostasis.

Mounting evidence suggests that a person's thoughts and feelings can influence the functioning of these systems, making us more... or less... susceptible to disease.

Most of us have developed certain operational restrictions that we use to keep us feeling safe in life. We maintain beliefs, experience a range of feeling states and entertain a range of thoughts that we interpret as "facts" or "true". These are personal interpretations and constraints whose value lies in helping us maintain equilibrium in a fast changing world. To be available for multiple perspectives isn't often practical and the uncertainty of such an existence is too frightening to maintain for long. However, some of these constraints may need to be temporarily unmasked in order to lift the underlying physiological restrictions if a cure is to be attempted.

Many aspects of life are so consistent and "matter of fact", that we regard them as irrefutable "facts". This makes life so much simpler. But when it comes to personal issues and beliefs, we may attribute the same surety to them when they are not so certain.

Our beliefs contribute to our feelings of safety and control, but they may also be making us biologically more rigid.

This lack of flexibility may be adversely affecting our capacity to respond fully and expansively to a threat to our own organism, confining our immune response and increasing our susceptibility to disease.

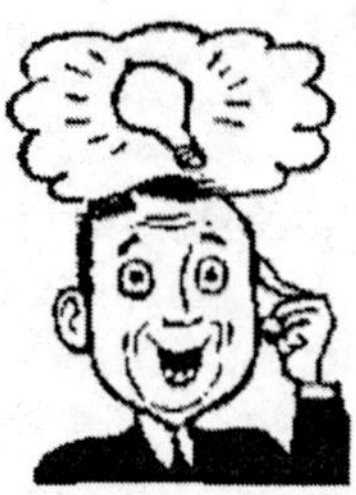

We're using defence mechanisms designed to protect us from circumstances which no longer exist, and as a consequence, our attempts to deal with current circumstances may be using mechanisms which are long out of date. We're responding to a present challenge using past responses.

The m3health Program is a way of unlocking the rigidity to which we've become accustomed. It requires of the inquirer that he opens his mind a little and becomes available for new realisations, new feelings, thoughts and perspectives. He'll need to be willing to experience the discomfort or fear of releasing old defences and risking incremental exposure to the unknown. His suffering may temporarily increase.

There's no point in replacing old rigidities with new ones. New beliefs held with the same rigidity as the old ones are not helpful. Coming to recognise that all thoughts and beliefs can potentially stop healing is a step forward. Understanding the implications of this takes time.

The m3health Program removes old restrictions to our beliefs, thoughts and feelings and restores our healing potential by freeing us to be more responsive.

Being more responsive means that our healing mechanisms can respond quicker, and more completely, to any external threat or to any internal imbalance.

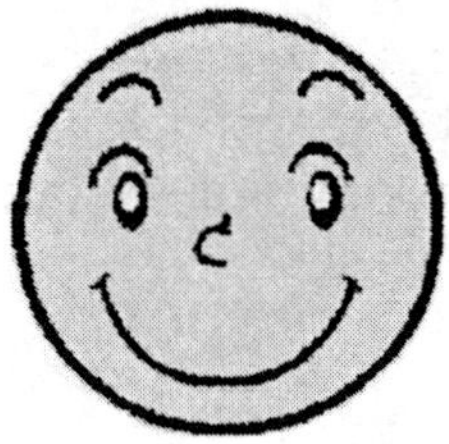

Undertaking the m3health Program begins the healing process.

8
ANONYMITY

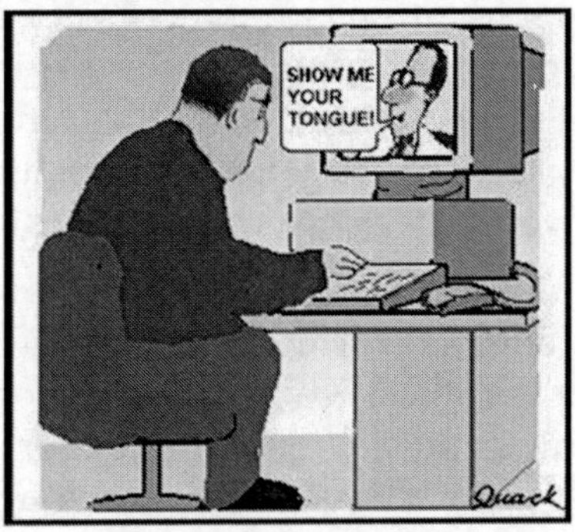

©Quack MD

If a doctor asks a patient "How often do you masturbate?"... the answer may be... "Once a fortnight". If a computer asks the same patient the same question the answer may be..... "Three times a week".

The m3health Program is undertaken by you, not your doctor. His role is important but different from yours.

The frequency with which you consult your usual medical attendant concerning your responses to the m3health Program is a matter concerning yourself and your doctor. You may have a good relationship with your health attendant which means that you discuss your responses with her. The purpose of your relationship with m3health is to improve your relationship with yourself. Your most vital relationship in your own healing is with yourself.

The subscriptions to further m3health options available on the website www.m3health.com may involve providing credit card information that may identify you. M3health is not privy to your identity nor personal details and will never send you anything other than information that you have specifically requested. We will respond only to the personal information that you provide in specific communications with us. The credit card information is a requirement of our payment processors and is not available to, nor of any interest to m3health.

We also offer alternative payment methods that provide an additional level of anonymity, should that be your choice.

M3health does not identify its convenors nor any of the parties responding to your communications as we believe that your interests are best served by you and us both remaining at arm's length, and for you to retain your relationship with your own medical advisors and enhance your relationship with yourself.

Medical authorities are not always aware of what the public wants, and new, effective forms of healing such as the m3health Program sometimes take a while to become established within the medical community. With your doctor's help you may need to do a bit of research yourself into your own problem.

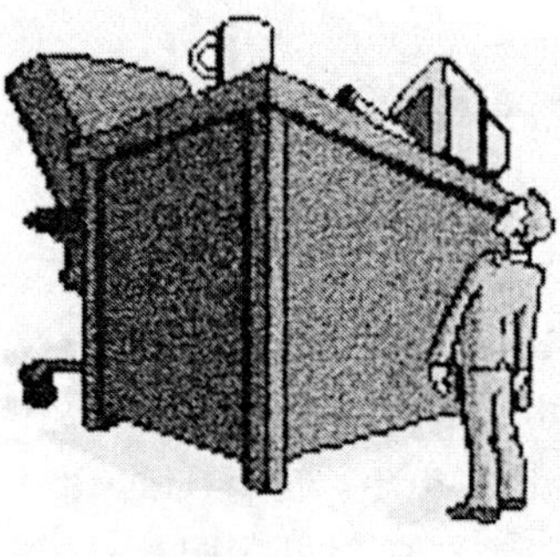

Your power to discern, and take responsibility for your decisions, is vital to your healing.

Your health may be better served by not handing responsibility to someone else, however competent and well meaning he or she may be, but by entering into a "health partnership" with your medical advisors.

9
DISCLAIMERS

PLEASE READ THIS CAREFULLY BEFORE YOU DECIDE TO UNDERTAKE THE M3HEALTH PROGRAM

The Health Partnership between a patient and his practitioner is an essential component of healing, providing the support for the patient to participate in the m3health Program.

This Program is intended for individuals who wish to assist the medical therapy that they're already undertaking, whether orthodox, alternative or complementary.

M3health has no opinion as to the suitability of treatments already undertaken by participants in the m3health Program, and is of the view that human biodiversity guarantees that some treatments work better for some people than for others, and work better at some times than at others.

M3health is of the view that orthodox medicine deserves to be investigated thoroughly and be given the opportunity to assist you.

The m3health Program is designed to be an adjunct to medical therapies and to be used concurrently with them. It is not to be used as a stand alone treatment for a medical condition.

The participant is encouraged to discuss any matter which arises in the course of the m3health Program with his medical attendant or with any other person, should he wish.

M3health encourages participants to undertake the Program in the spirit in which the convenors intended it be undertaken. This book is an ethical and serious attempt to improve the health and the life of each and every participant. M3health believes that this is self-evident on any reading of the material.

M3health requests that if it's unlikely you'll allow m3health to be of value to yourself at this time, then you do not continue with the m3health Program.

If this is not the right time for you to explore the origins of your disease and possible remedies, m3health is unlikely to be of assistance to you at this time. You may elect to come back to it later.

It is expressly acknowledged by m3health that uncomfortable feelings and thoughts arise in the course of any true exploration, and at these times participants may want to consult with their doctor and perhaps discuss engaging a face to face therapist, or seek other assistance. M3health leaves that decision up to the participants.

FOR PARTICIPANTS IN THE M3HEALTH PROGRAM

I agree to take personal responsibility for participating in the m3health Program.

I agree that I, and others acting on my behalf, will not hold m3health responsible for my suffering.

FROM OUR LEGAL PEOPLE: INDEMNITY

You agree to defend, indemnify, and hold Runfox Pty Ltd., its officers, directors, employees, agents, licensors, and suppliers, harmless from and against any claims, actions or demands, liabilities and settlements including without limitation, reasonable legal and accounting fees, resulting from, or alleged to result from, your violation of these Terms and Conditions.

Section 3: The m3health Program

The Open Road

Summary of m3health Program Chapters

1. First Step	A thorough evaluation of your current therapy.
2. Your Family	Beliefs and attitudes acquired within the family may be inhibiting our healing potential.
3. Illness confirms beliefs	We say "Life sucks!" because we're ill. However, we may be ill because we already believe "Life sucks!"
4. Who am I?	What has our personality got to do with our illness and our recovery from it?
5. Responses to being ill	Illness is emotive. It provides a powerful opportunity to unmask thoughts and feelings that have remained hidden for a long time and may be keeping you ill.
6. Glossary of Terms	The origin of terms such as "dis-ease", "re-present", "respons-ibility" are discussed and the contribution an understanding of them makes to both the origins of, and the recovery from, illness.
7. Knowledge	How what you "know" may be stopping you from recovering. Read the last sentence again. Did you understand it the first time?

8. First nature and second nature — We're all familiar with the term "second nature" without ever considering that it implies the existence of "first nature". What is first nature and how can we involve it in our own healing?

9. The immune system — How our thoughts and feelings limit our natural responses.

10. Thoughts — One of the most powerful causes of pain and suffering comes from our thoughts. We need to use this powerful force, but not by trying to change what we think, and certainly not by replacing "negative" thoughts with "positive" thoughts, but by allowing all thoughts to visit us.......and to leave us. Stop thinking and allow yourself to be "thunk".

11. Feelings — The four basic emotions of anger, sadness, fear and joy and their integral relationship to the proper functioning of our immune and endocrine (hormonal) systems.

12. Express or Repress — The effect on our health of repressing emotions and what happens when we take the risk of expressing them.

13. Anger — Does it deserve its bad press? What's the difference between anger and violence? Can we use healthy anger to assist healing?

14. Practising Feeling Emotions — Unlocking feelings to unlock the immune and endocrine systems.

15. Fear — At the bottom of many an illness. Anxiety and panic unmasked.

16. Sadness	Usually more of a problem with men. It's important to involve the full range of physiological responses, such as crying, in an m3health Program of recovery.
17. Joy	Putting joy back into life with laughter and love.
18. The Feral Healer	Unleashing an old friend to help you.
19. Half-way review	A review of the journey thus far.
20. Moving Right Along	Taking your time.
21. Doing	The obsession with "doing" may be restricting your healing.
22. Et tu Bruté?	Are we are our worst enemy when it comes to getting better?
23. Cause and Cure	The forgotten origins of illness and the ignored main healing element.
24. Self Acceptance	Why we criticise ourselves and how we might use that realisation to move on.
25. Judgement	The decommissioning of the prime mover of chronic dis-ease.
26. Being	Most of us have forgotten how to "be". Being isn't lost, only hidden. We may need to re-experience it to heal ourselves.
27. Self	At the core of our healing nature or first nature lies an untapped resource.
28. Meditation	Practising doing *nothing* so that your body can achieve *something*.

29. Finding our Selfs — Hiding under the canopy of our defences is something we mislaid, rather than lost. We "find ourselves" doing, thinking and feeling.....something.....it doesn't matter much what. Find your "self" and healing won't be far behind.

30. Acceptance — Accepting ourselves, whoever, whenever, however, wherever we are. What does this involve? Is it something that you "**Do**"?

31. Letting Go — Not something that you *do*, but something that shows up.

32. Control — *"You're out of control"* becomes music to your ears when you realise the cost of staying *"In control"*.

33. Guilt, Fault and Blame — These powerful emotions often contribute to illness and must be harnessed for healing.

34. Should and Ought — Remember these. How do we know what's best for us? Perhaps we don't. Then how do we know what we "should" be doing or what we "ought" to have done?

1
First Step

Welcome to the m3heath Program, your Highway to Health.

Firstly, we need a thorough evaluation of the current illness.

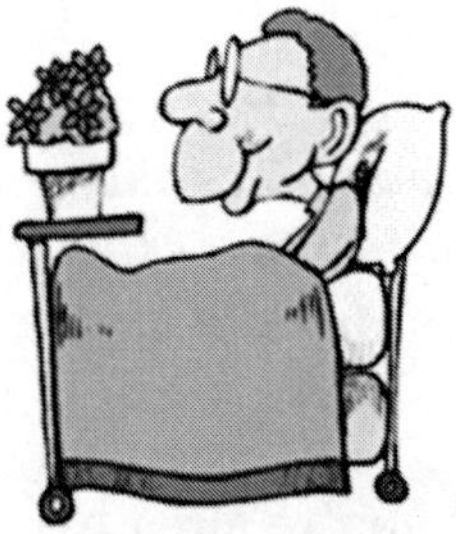

If serious illness has been longstanding, medical specialists find it difficult looking at the condition with fresh eyes. They're often guided by what they themselves have previously thought about the problem or have been given a pre-conceived diagnosis by someone else, usually the referring doctor or the patient. It's quite hard getting someone to look at the problem from a fresh perspective — to start with a clean slate.

Patients must assist here by playing their part in their own recovery. In today's medico-legal climate their doctor is not at liberty to go beyond the "known". His role may be to support his patient, to encourage him to inquire, and for the patient to return to discuss what he's found.

The natural timeframe to establish a diagnosis may be months or even years, and if a diligent doctor remains persistent and committed, a good result can be obtained.

So gather all the information about your illness, including the existing opinions on how to proceed, and ask yourself whether you've exhausted all avenues that have been recommended to you in which you still retain some faith. If some of these remain unexplored or incompletely explored, orthodox or alternative, consider whether you need to take steps to complete those recommendations. As mentioned previously, it can take years in some instances for a diagnosis to be made upon which effective treatment can be based.

> ***Remember the idea of a "health partnership" in which you and your medical advisors play complementary roles. The practitioner brings medical knowledge to the exercise and you bring yourself, with your often intuitive and medically "unscientific" views about how to proceed. But of course you bring much more than that. Your investment in a good outcome cannot be purchased nor assigned to someone else, however well meaning and however qualified.***

The m3health Program is intended to be used in conjunction with any therapy that you're already undertaking or about to undertake. So you can begin the m3health Program even if you have unfinished medical recommendations to complete.

> ***During the m3health Program, we will concern ourselves less with the conventional view of the disease and more with the person suffering from it.***

Please introduce yourself.

Thank you. Now in responding to the following questions you may have an immediate answer followed by a more reflective response. Allow both to arise and take your time, remembering that the m3health Program has no timeframe and no "right" answers. Note what emotions arise in answering the questions. I use the word "answer" as it's commonly used, but the better word is "response". You need not "answer" the questions in the sense of reaching a conclusion, but rather "respond" to them. They will initiate a response in you. Those responses will consist of doing, thinking and feeling. The four basic feelings are anger, sadness, fear and joy. We will consider them in detail later.

Some people like to make notes, write out their thoughts, record them on tape, video themselves or have another person present. Feel free to use any methodology that appeals to you. The website www.m3health.com provides both an electronic log, m3diary, and an assessment tool, m3checkit, to assist you. Reports on your personal progress are available by subscribing to an m3 personal report, available on the website on the *subscription information* page.

One of the advantages in recording your responses is to check them later or show them to others whose observations you value. Listening or watching yourself speak about yourself can be a valuable experience, revealing hidden attitudes and responses. Many of these questions may not appear to have a direct relationship with your state of health.

- Are you in a relationship?
- Do you have any children?

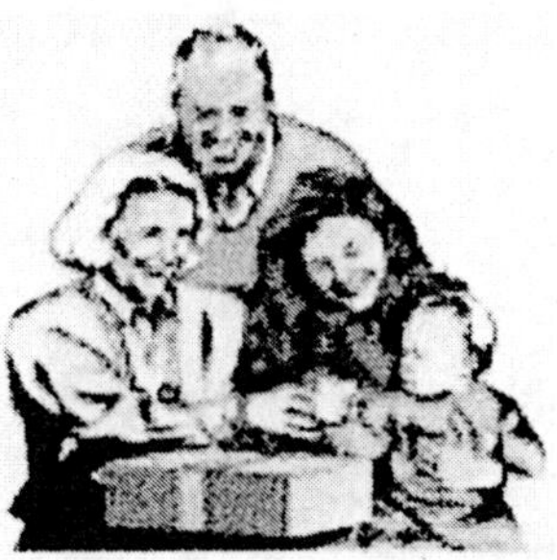

- Have you any brothers or sisters?
- Are your parents still alive?
- Have any of your own children died?
- How are you getting on in your relationship?
- Has there been a change in your relationship because of an illness?
- Is there any part of that change that pleases you?

- What's your partner's response to your illness?
- Are you familiar with that response in your life?

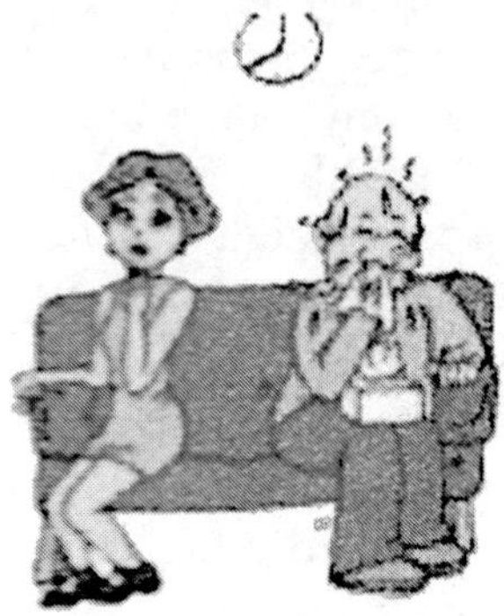

- Have you experienced people responding to you in a similar manner before?
- Who was that and when was it?

2
YOUR FAMILY

Most of us have two families:

(a) Our immediate family made up of our partners and our children

(b) Our original family in which we grew up

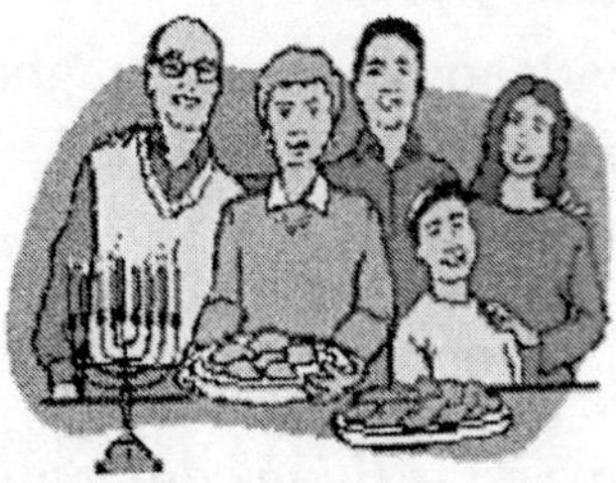

The family in which we grew up is usually accredited with those values and attitudes that we carry from childhood into adult life. We may have complied with them or rebelled against them, but either way they may still be influencing a substantial proportion of our thoughts, feelings and actions, i.e. our responses. This means that instead of being free to respond to a stimulus in the present, our response is dictated to some degree by old attitudes. Our physiology may be equally restricted, responding out of the past and not in the present, resulting in illness. To recover we may need to explore some of these restrictions. They may firstly need to be uncovered, since we've lived with them so long they've become "second nature", and we're often unaware of them. Let's uncover some of them.

- What do you say about yourself?

Take your time with this question. A flippant response is itself significant, and underneath it, if you're prepared to acknowledge your flippancy, will often be some fairly heavily defended beliefs about you, rarely admitted to yourself or to anyone else. The beginning of illness is also rarely brought into awareness until the symptoms become increasingly difficult to ignore.

- What statements could you make with some certainty about life?

It could be helpful here to write these down at this early stage of your personal exploration, as it can be of interest to revisit them later.

We're often critical of our self, others, or more commonly....... both.

- Do you criticise yourself?

Are you familiar with any of these thoughts:

"There's something wrong with me"

"I should be better"

"I'm hopeless"

"I ought to have done things differently"

"I'm not good enough"

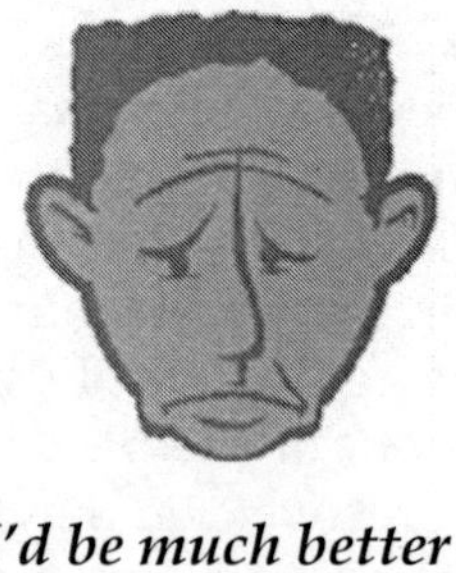

"If only...............I'd be much better off"

"I ought to have gotten over this by now"

"Why can't I...."

"I'm bad"

"I should be able to...."

"What's the matter with me?"

"I ought to be different."

Or perhaps you don't criticise yourself much but tend to criticise others.

- Are you familiar with the thoughts, expressed or otherwise....

"I'm better than anyone else"

"If you want it done you have to do it yourself"

"You just can't trust anyone"

"They're just no damn good"

"Why must I always have to do it myself"

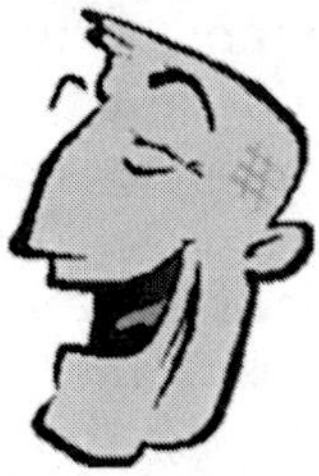

"People generally piss me off"

"There's nothing wrong with me, it's him/her/them who's hopeless"

"You can count the number of people of calibre that you'll meet in life on the fingers of one hand"

"Most employees are pretty bloody useless when it comes to it"

Or you may find yourself complaining to the Universe

"Why me? Why does it always have to be me!"

"Why can't someone else suffer for a while!"

"What have I ever done to anyone!"

"What have I done to deserve this!"

"Someone out there's really got it in for me!"

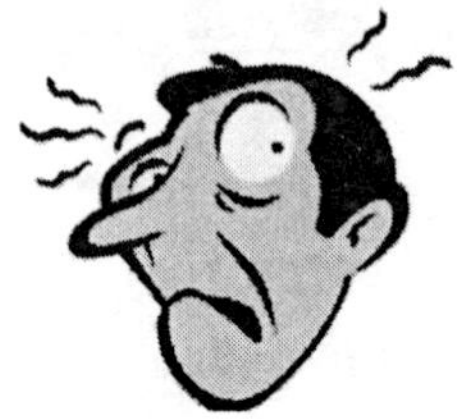

Much of what we regard as the "truth" is not an objective distillation of available evidence but what we've been taught or have deduced from the narrow perspective of our personal experience.

The beliefs we adopt enable us to live less complicated lives, filter unwanted stimuli and defuse difficult subjects. We congregate with people of similar beliefs for ease and safety. Most of these beliefs cause us no harm and in fact help us through life, enabling us to belong. However, if we're suffering from chronic or serious illness, some of those same beliefs that have helped us in the past may now be harming us. We may need to broaden our horizons, putting aside old prejudices and judgements and allowing ourselves new perspectives. Because we've adopted our attitudes, beliefs and "truths" for protection, i.e. to feel safe and cared for as children, we're reluctant to give them up now as grownups, however damaging they're proving to be. We like to see them as universal truths, not as beliefs peculiar to our community and ourselves. It's hard to acknowledge that they may have outlived their usefulness. It's hard to believe that they're not universally true but convenient fictions.

A good example of "truths" in perspective is the multiple religious conflicts taking place all over the world, with proponents from both sides equally convinced of the righteousness and truth of their positions, never stopping to consider that had they been born a short distance away they may well be fighting with equal conviction for their sworn enemies.

There's no point replacing the old beliefs with a new, equally restrictive set, or replace one set of fictions with a new set of fictions. It may be more beneficial to explore the nature of all beliefs, whatever they may be. That way we enter into a different relationship with our beliefs...... you could say that they no longer run us.

Let's consider the ramifications of some of the beliefs we hold dear.

It doesn't matter what the actual belief is. "I'm truly hopeless", or "I'm simply the best". They are both equally restrictive of healing.

> ***The <u>conviction</u> with which the belief was adopted in the first place, and the <u>need to defend it</u> thereafter, are the energies that inhibit the body's healing capabilities.***
>
> ***The actual belief itself is irrelevant.***

The critical thing at this point of our m3health Program is to simply become aware that the thoughts we have are not "true".

Most of the time we're even unaware that we're actually thinking.

We relate to the thoughts running through our minds as if they are "reality", whereas they're actually a response of ours to a stimulus. No two human beings, given an identical stimulus, have an identical response, because no two of us have had the same upbringing and experience and hence our natures differ and the filters (defences) that create our "realities" differ.

The following sequence of events results in thoughts, feelings and actions.

We monitor our environment using our senses; sight, hearing, taste, smell and touch.

We respond to the environmental stimuli registered by our senses.

Those responses include thoughts, feelings and actions.

We're usually aware that we're ***doing*** something, and sometimes that we're ***feeling*** something, but often not that we're ***thinking*** something.

To become aware that

"we are thinking"

is a giant leap towards freedom

from those thoughts.

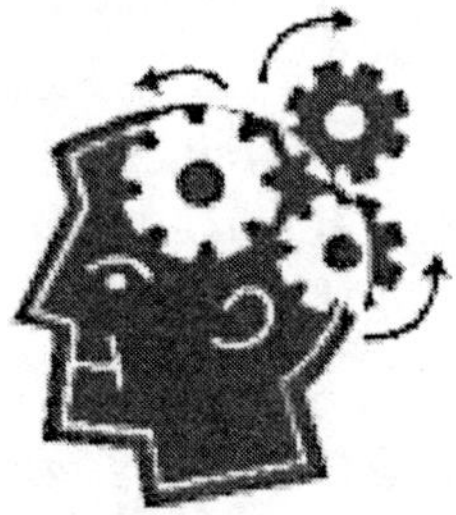

It places a "watcher" between the thinker and his thoughts.

3
Illness Confirms Beliefs

How do we use our responses to free ourselves from disease?

Recall that a chronic problem may be "re-presenting" an unresolved issue. The issue is being brought into the present, i.e. re-present-ed. The old problem circulates, trapped within our minds and bodies, directing us towards a set of present circumstances in which it has a chance to both prove itself and also resolve itself. We locate ourselves within these circumstances so that healing can happen. We gravitate towards the conditions. This is part of our biological heritage in which the body and mind are always trying to heal us. We don't usually determine these things consciously.

Take our thoughts about illness.

We believe that we're thinking certain thoughts because we're ill, but the reverse may be the case. We may be ill because we're thinking that way.

One such thought might be "Life sucks!" We claim we think "Life sucks!" because we're ill. However, it may not be the illness which makes us think "life sucks!" Maybe we think "life sucks!" anyway...already...and the illness merely confirms our belief. We've gravitated towards illness for two reasons.

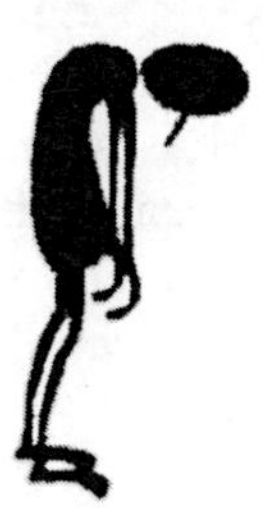

The first is that the illness confirms what we already believe, thereby keeping life within the boundaries of the "known", and therefore safe, though more painful. The second reason is that the suffering gives us an incentive to take corrective action.

To take it a step further, we're attracted to the illness because it brings to the surface our existing but perhaps buried belief that "life sucks". If the illness didn't create that thought, then what did? For the answer to that we need to go back to a time when we were formulating our beliefs about ourselves, and life generally.

Let's continue to use the belief that "life sucks" as our example.

When was it that you first came across that belief? Did someone you know have that belief, or behaved as if they did? Was that person either your mother or your father? If it was either parent, can you acknowledge the possibility that you don't believe that "life sucks" because of your current illness, but that you already believe it from childhood?

A belief that "life sucks" may not be conducive to good health. It may lead to despondency, despair and eventually to destitution. It stops you feeling joy and may modify your capacity to express anger, sadness and fear, perhaps replacing them with depression. It changes the body physiology and may, over time, lead to disease. Now here's the really important thing about beliefs.

Any belief, rigidly held, restricts our view. It equally restricts the body physiology, limiting the capacity of those systems to heal us.

The belief that "life sucks" is neither true nor untrue. It's simply a belief that you picked up as a child. And it's very powerful because the child has no additional perspective from which to argue against it. Because this belief is nagging away inside you and you may be unaware of it, you may be attracted to circumstances in which you can declare it to be true, such as serious illness. The illness serves to confirm the belief.

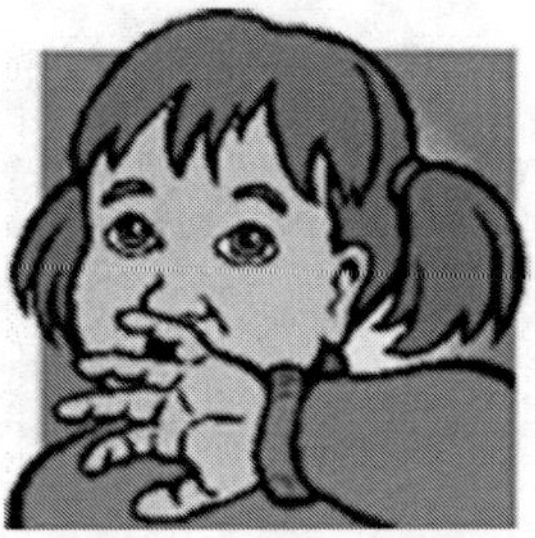

But why would anyone want a negative belief to be confirmed?

We adopted that belief in childhood in order to conform with the beliefs of those people around us, parents usually, who kept us alive. For safety we had little option but to concur with either what was being told to us directly or what was modelled or implied to us. As adults we're attracted to, or create circumstances in which we get to re-experience those old beliefs, however damaging, in order to feel safe.

We prefer the pain of the known to the fear of the unknown.

Now here's the good part!

The contemporary circumstances to which we're attracted in order to confirm the old beliefs and stay safe also brings those beliefs, and their associated suffering, to the surface, i.e. into consciousness. If we're prepared to take a risk and explore them, realising eventually that they're neither true nor untrue – they're what we've been taught as children – we can use this current episode to move beyond the original belief.

How do we do that?

We don't have to "do" anything.

It's already happening.

We simply continue the exploration.

4

WHO AM I?

The following questions mobilise thoughts and feelings.

They raise into consciousness long-standing unfinished business which contributes to disease. We're stirring the pot here a little, providing an opportunity for anything requiring attention to percolate to the top.

We'll consider possible responses later, and what they might be pointing towards. For the time being just allow anything which surfaces to do so.

There's no right way of doing this.

- Are you in a relationship?

Let's use this simple question to explore undertaking the m3health Program in a beneficial rather than a superficial way.

There's the simple "yes" or "no" answer to this question, which, since we already "know" the answer, takes us nowhere.

Then there's the "allowing whatever comes up" methodology.

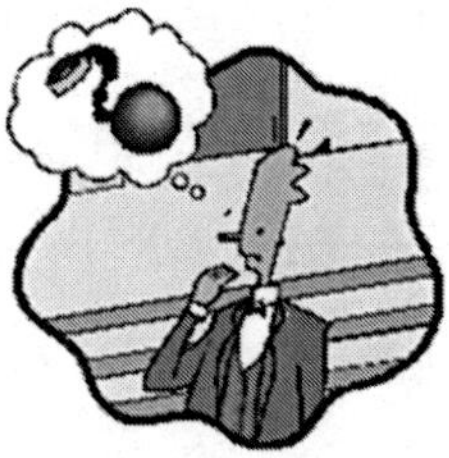

Very few people can think about their relationship or lack of one without feeling something. If we give ourselves the time, then multiple images, thoughts, beliefs, feelings, bodily sensations and perhaps even actions will reach consciousness from this simple question alone. The business of life has not permitted these to surface previously, but now our commitment to the m3health Program is such that we allow them to surface. In so doing the origin of our beliefs about our relationship may be revealed.

If I believe "my husband's untrustworthy", is it because he is untrustworthy, or do I believe "he's untrustworthy" in order to keep faith with my mother's belief about men? Is this in my best interests? Do I need my husband to be untrustworthy just so that I can re-affirm my long-standing belief? Am I pushing him towards other women in order to prove myself right? What other beliefs do I hold about men which come into this category, i.e. beliefs which I regurgitate by rote whilst insisting that they're independent, objective beliefs? What does "trusting" him mean anyway? Am I making him responsible for my happiness by claiming that if he's not trustworthy, then I can't be happy? If that's the case, why do I need to be unhappy? Who told me that life was a place in which one should only expect unhappiness? What else in my life am I using to confirm this particular belief? Whoops.......could this be the reason for the recurring bronchitis from which I'm suffering? Wow! I've just realised that if I get healthy I'll have to stop blaming him for everything. Now that will be scary!! Hmmmm...maybe the bronchitis isn't so bad after all.......

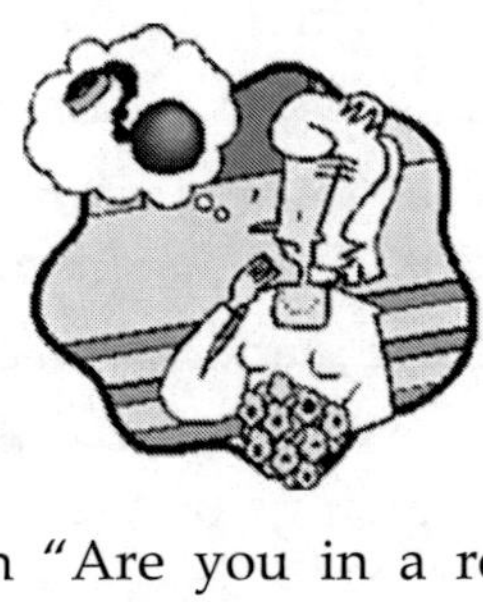

The simple question "Are you in a relationship?" spawns multiple questions and responses.

Let's continue....

- Do you have any children?
- Have you any brothers or sisters?

- Are your parents still alive?
- Have any of your loved ones died?
- How are you getting on in your relationship?
- Has there been a change in your relationship because of the illness?
- Is there any part of that change which pleases you?
- What is your partner's response to your illness?
- Are you familiar with that response in your life?
- Who in your life previously had a similar response and when was it?
- Are you lonely?

  If your answer to this question is emphatic, either an emphatic "yes" or an emphatic "no", then your answer contains energy. Follow the energy trail by making your answer even more emphatic for a while. Yell out loud "I am not lonely", or "I'm lonely" and allow the underlying emotions to rise to the surface. Then be quiet for a while.

  Accentuating the emotional component reduces the analytical thinking that we may be using to suppress what we're really feeling.
- Is this illness helpful in some way?
- How would you like your personal life to be different?
- Does this illness get you any caring or consideration you weren't previously getting and wanted?
- Is the illness making matters worse?
- Is there someone in your life; partner, parents, children, friends who isn't giving you the respect and caring you want from him or her?
- Is there any secret in your life which is a burden to you?
- Apart from being rid of this illness, what do you want to be different in your life?

Was your response, "Nothing!" "I just want to be rid of this disease, that's all!"

Did you feel anger?

Is anger a common feeling for you since you developed this disease?

Has it really annoyed or irritated you when people imply that you're not trying to get well?

Have you had the response "Well, what would they know!"

Is there something about you which no-one or hardly anyone knows?

- Are you hurting about something?
- Is life tough?
- Do you silently weep?

At the end of responding to the above questions, perhaps you could give yourself a little time to do nothing but be with yourself. Take note of whether that appeals to you, or whether you find other matters too pressing. If that's the case, perhaps you could consciously decide to come back to yourself when you have a moment.

take it EASY

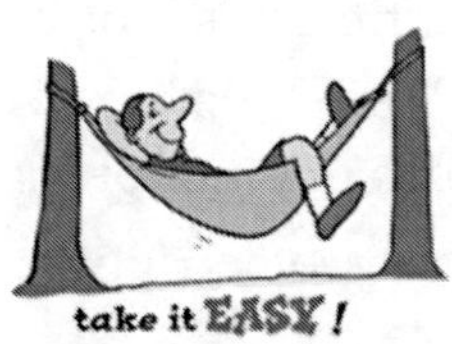

If you do have the time to spend with yourself now, let whatever thoughts and feelings arise just be there. No treatment, no therapy, no analysis of them is required. They require no justification and there may be no "good" reason for them being there.

Notice whether there were more thoughts than feelings or vice versa. Are you more comfortable with thinking about things than feeling things, you might ask yourself.

Either way, are you able to accept whatever your responses were, and yourself for having them?

5
RESPONSES

Illness is emotive.

Allow any thoughts and feelings to arise whilst you're going through the following questions. There may be some discomfort from old impasses coming to the surface again. If the process becomes too uncomfortable: Stop. Come back to it later when you're ready. Later might be minutes or years, later. You can always discuss your responses friends, family, or with your medical attendant.

I use the notion of four basic feelings states — anger, sadness, fear and joy. More complex but common feelings are a mixture of the above, such as guilt, anxiety, blame, humiliation, etc. Other commentators differentiate between feelings and emotions and have a different set of basic feelings. It doesn't matter which framework you use.

We'll focus upon feelings or emotions later.

With the questions there are no right or wrong answers. Take your time.

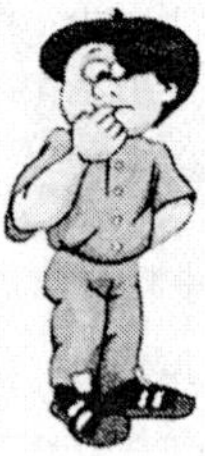

- What's the most common thought you've had whilst trying to get rid of this disease?
- Is that a thought with which you're familiar?
- Where did it come from do you think?

- Has anyone else in your family suffered in a similar manner?
- Have you had other episodes of illness or problems in your life during which you experienced similar thoughts and feelings?

  Make a careful note of the circumstances in which you found yourself at those times.
- Can you remember if either of your parents or important caregivers had similar beliefs and feelings to the ones that you're expressing now?

What were they?

Take your time over this question because parental attitudes are not often out in the open and the child doesn't think like an adult. You may have to deduce parental attitudes from your observations as an older child, even though younger children are generally more responsive to parental attitudes than older ones.

Let's now focus upon changes in your life at the time of this illness.

- What's changed in your life as a consequence of being ill?

  List both "bad" and "good" consequences.
- Did you have a response to the suggestion that some good may have come from being ill?
- What was that response?
- Are you familiar with it?
- Have you received more or less caring since being ill?

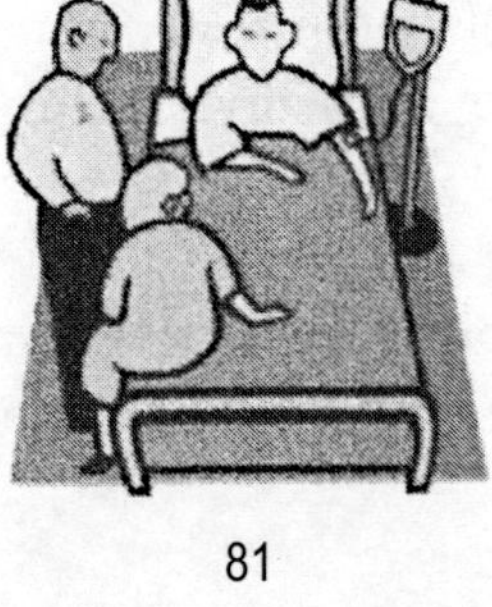

- Whose attitude to you has changed?
- How has it changed?
- What has been your response to the caring you receive as a consequence of being ill?
- What attitudes to love and caring have been "confirmed" from being ill?
- Where did those attitudes come from?
- Are you suffering in silence?
- Which person(s) do you want to become aware of the real extent of your suffering?
- What do you say to yourself about the degree to which you should make others aware of your suffering?
- Who does this remind you of?
- Is "being strong" important to you?

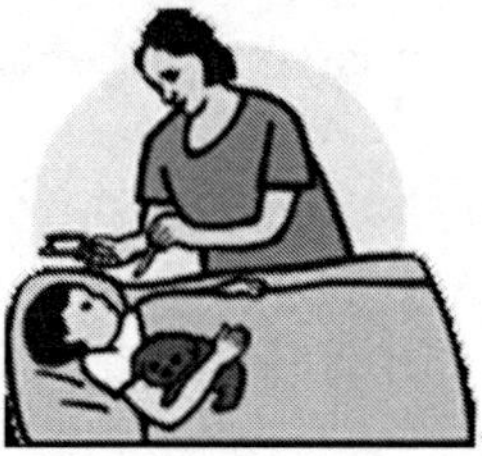

- Did you have to be strong as a child?

  Why?
- Does this illness enable you to take care of someone else better than you would otherwise have done?

In other words, are you taking care of someone else's needs by being ill?

Whose?

Has this happened before?

By being ill are you attracting caring which is otherwise unavailable to you?

Who's providing that additional caring?

- What do you think about people who are always ill?
- Are you aware of anyone else in your life with similar beliefs?

- Is this illness preventing you from accomplishing something?

Complete the following: "If it weren't for this illness I'd................"

Would you be frightened to achieve this on some level?

Are you afraid that if you weren't ill that you'd be expected to do something you're apprehensive about?

Who would expect that of you?

- Did you suffer from diarrhoea or asthma as a kid when you had to do something scary, like exams or sport?
- Were there any other childhood illnesses from which you suffered, on reflection, because you were expected to achieve something?
- Who had these expectations of you?
- Who were you expected to impress, or wanted to impress?
- Were either of your parents, doctors, nurses, social workers, psychologists or from any other of the helping professions?
- What was his or her general attitude to illness?
- Who got most caring in your family?

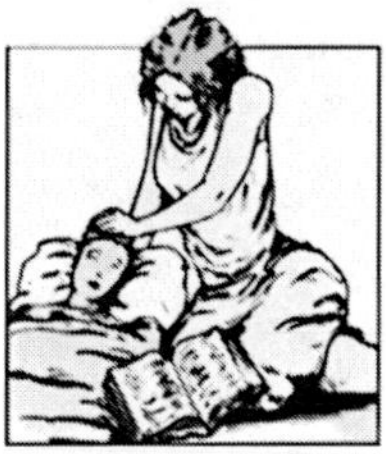

From whom?

Why?

What feelings have you been having since becoming ill?

The basic feelings are anger (irritable, annoyed, pissed off, frustrated), sadness (weepy, blue, down), fear (scared, frightened, apprehensive, worried, anxious) or joy (happy, blissful, carefree).

- Are you unhappy?

  With what?

  With whom?
- Do you curse this illness?

  What do you say?

  If you were to curse someone else in a way similar to the way in which you're cursing this illness, who might that be?
- Do you curse yourself in a way similar to the way in which you find yourself cursing this illness?
- How long have you been doing that for?
- Does it annoy you when people imply that you're to blame for this illness in some way?
- Do you blame yourself for the illness?
- Do you blame yourself for anything else?
- Are you hurting inside?

At the end of responding to the above questions, perhaps you could give yourself a little time to do nothing but be with yourself. Take note of whether that appeals to you, or whether you find other matters pressing upon you that you must take care of. If that's the case, perhaps you could decide to come back to yourself when you have a moment. If you do have the time to spend with yourself now, let whatever thoughts and feelings arise just be there.

No treatment, no therapy, no analysis of them is required.

They require no justification and there may be no "good" reason for having them.

Once again, notice whether there were more thoughts than feelings, or vice versa.

- "Am I more comfortable with thinking about things than feeling things", you might wonder aloud.
- Either way, are you able to accept yourself and your responses, or are you annoyed with yourself?

O.K. That's fine.

6
Words and Their Meanings

The words we use often contain hidden or forgotten meanings.

More recent interpretations of words often imply meanings which contain more certainty or safety than the original meaning. It can be helpful in our inquiry to look back to the original structure of the word. Living with uncertainty might be a more natural state than imagining certainty where none really exists. Some of these terms follow.

REPRESENT

The current illness often represents something from the past.

The present component of the word needs to be pronounced as in the phrase "present time". Present is itself comprised of "Pre" and "sent", i.e. it has been sent before. Re-present means to take something from the past and to bring it into the present time. Please take as long as you need to make this connection, as it makes much of the m3health Program self-evident. Without fully and comprehensively understanding the origin of the word "represent", it's difficult to understand the basic mechanism of illness creation. The current circumstances are representative of past, unfinished business, and provide an opportunity for completion in the present. An acute (current) illness may become chronic (long-term) because the immune system is not functioning sufficiently well to combat it. The old unresolved issue may be diminishing the effectiveness of the immune system.

The individual is attracted to present circumstances which bear some relationship to unfinished business because they hold the potential to resolve the old issue, i.e. they can re-*present* it or bring it into the here and now.

Evolution demands that the body and mind try and heal themselves. Because of this the organism (us) is attracted to circumstances capable of assisting with healing.

RESPONSE

We react to external stimuli with a response.

The response consists of actions, thoughts and feelings. The basic four feeling states are anger, sadness, fear and joy.

The m3health Program initiates a response that we can observe. We can assess how mechanical and rigid our responses may have become over time.

The mind and body are healthier if they can respond freely to a threat.

The freeing of our responses *is* the healing process.

RESPONSIBILITY

To understand the meaning we assign to this word we can use the French spelling, responsabilitie. In English response-ibility is derived from response-ability, i.e. the *ability to respond.*

SELF "RESPONS-ABILITY"

Self-responsibility is the cornerstone of healing, for without it we continue to act as children, not responding unfettered to present circumstances but with responses dictated by old, leftover adaptations. Some of those adaptations have restricted our capacity for healing.

To take responsibility means being willing to explore our responses. This continues for our entire adult life and frees our healing response.

It always involves some fear, often experienced as excitement, and perhaps even fun.

INQUIRY OR ENQUIRY

To inquire is to look with new eyes and not with one's mind already made up about "how things are". In the m3health Program, certainty is replaced by uncertainty. Certainty demands that matters be "known", and the denial of doubt, in an attempt to remain comfortable, or avoid fear. Uncertainty acknowledges that healing may lie beyond "knowing". Inquiring allows another energy to arise in the void created by the departure of certainty.

SUFFER

Suffering is the experience of emotions, thoughts, and perhaps bodily sensations that we don't like. It implies some resistance to these experiences.

If the emotions, thoughts and sensations are allowed, without interference and without resistance, would suffering continue?

Moving from suffering to acceptance may be a matter of allowing ourselves to feel fear. We're often afraid to experience fear.

Because few of us are capable of present time responses, we suffer when we're ill and when we're frightened of an undesirable outcome. Suffering may occur when we move from the known to the unknown. The degree of suffering is proportional to the degree of resistance to thinking, feeling and acting spontaneously. There's a difference between being spontaneous and being precipitous. The former implies a natural unfettered response, the latter a response dictated by the need to complete the matter before running its natural course. This is usually an attempt to diminish the sensation of fear.

DISEASE

Disease means dis-ease, un-easy or dis-comfort.

ACUTE

An acute illness comes and goes quickly. Because the body has resolved the disease (often despite the treatment we've administered), no m3health Program is necessary. If multiple acute episodes occur which begin to interfere with our enjoyment of life we may be prepared to look at what role we can play in preventing a recurrence.

CHRONIC

A chronic illness is one that goes on and on, seems not to be responding to treatment, and probably has an underlying component to which we're contributing. The disease is an expression of an underlying "dis-ease", or discomfort, an unresolved energy creating a longer term change in our physiology.

Some commentators claim that to cure long-standing illness, one needs to convert a chronic illness into an acute illness. This is why we go searching for a set of circumstances capable of bringing the physiological and psychological components of the original "dis-ease" to the surface, where they can be accessed more readily.

BECAUSE

Broken down into "be the cause" of, *because* is one of the most commonly used terms in English. It implies that something, often one thing, is the "cause" of another. Almost invariably, the cause ascribed to any event is incomplete or fallacious. The nominated "cause" may indeed be a "contributing factor", but is rarely, if ever, the one and only factor. Most statements containing the word "because" are usually expedient and self-serving, including any statements which I may make in this book *because* I'm trying to make a point. Perhaps we'd all be better served if I said that I don't really know why I'm making claims, but that I'd found the m3health Program to be of assistance with people's problems and don't really understand why. ☺

UNDERSTAND

M3health sometimes uses the term "understand". As an inquiry does not demand any conclusions, it is not the intention that an understanding of a matter concludes it. If we remain available for our views to mature with experience, our immune and endocrine systems are best positioned to respond immediately and effectively to any challenge to our organism.

Our relationship with all other living organisms is also maturing as both we, and they, evolve. Those organisms include other people and animals, but equally importantly, the billions of bacteria, viruses and other organisms which also inhabit our physical form, primarily on the surface of our body and within our gut.

"Understanding" therefore implies an evolving appreciation, rather than a finite and closed knowledge.

7
KNOWLEDGE

Firstly we need to find out what we "know". Much of the time we take things for granted, mistaking opinion for fact.

The immune system might benefit from removing the shackles imposed upon it by "the known", the "facts" and "certainty".

The more certain an opinion, the more unreliable it is!

Even that opinion, like all others, is unreliable. And that one also etc....etc.

Of many things we can be pretty certain, though never 100% sure, such as the sun will rise tomorrow morning. Many "facts" serve us well and will not be the subject of our m3health Program. However, some of what we've accepted for the sake of safety is now a liability rather than an asset. This is particularly so for those things we've come to accept as truth, reality or fact in the area of our personal beliefs. We may be better served if we restore these things to their position of "helpful expediencies". Then we can enter into a different relationship with them, be less dependent on them, and less restricted by them.

> The m3health Program is not aiming to increase my pool of knowledge, but instead it provides me with an opportunity to escape the restraints of what I already "know"

How is knowledge acquired?

We all have a set of utterly individual experiences as we travel through our lives, and these experiences over time become knowledge. Since everyone's journey is different, we all acquire a different knowledge set, i.e. know different things. And so not all knowledge is universal, leaving a lot of scope for people to argue over the "facts".

As modern physics and astronomy toil with the notions of multiple parallel universes, so the biological sciences acknowledge that the universe of every single organism is different.

We can only experience a fraction of what's available to be experienced. Nobody to date has experienced being on Mars, but one day someone most likely will. So our knowledge is at best a fraction of that available. We could group knowledge into several categories.

1. What we, "know that we know". (KK)
2. What we, "know that we don't know". (KDK)
3. What we, "don't know that we know". (DKK)
4. What we, "don't know that we don't know". (DKDK)

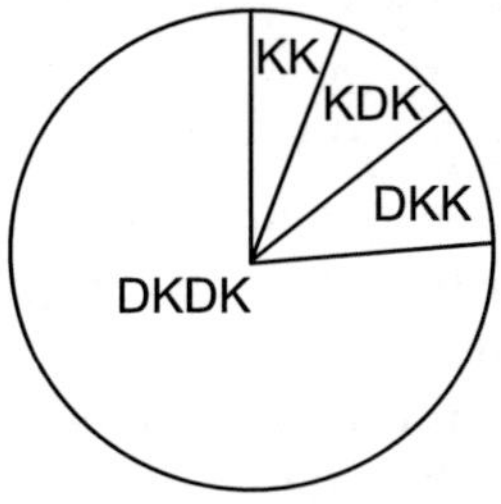

What we *know that we know* would include knowing your own name. You know that you know it.

What we *know that we don't know* could include the time of high tide for the day. We know that it's knowable, but we just don't happen to have that information right now.

What we *don't know that we know* could include subconsciously acquired information or intuitive information that cannot be brought into consciousness.

What we *don't know that we don't know* includes an area of knowledge we haven't come across before, so we're unaware of anything knowable or unknowable in that field. Most of what is potentially knowable is probably in this category.

What is experience?

Our five senses register sight, sound, touch, smell and taste, and together they build our experience. These senses are themselves limited, so that an owl has a different appreciation of the universe from a fish or from ourselves. In the case of the sense of sight, we can only see the "visible spectrum": red, orange, yellow, green, blue, indigo and violet. We can't see any wavelength of light shorter than violet, i.e. ultraviolet, and we can't see any wavelength longer than red, i.e. infrared. The light spectrum available to us is extremely limited. So we come to know only those things that we can see and those limited experiences become the basis of the known. The same limitations apply to the other senses as well.

Hmmmmm... "I'll believe that when I see it!".... I hear you murmuring.

The next matter to consider in our attempt to explore the nature of what we believe we "know" is to consider one of the senses. Once again let's use the sense of sight.

We believe that we see things with our eyes, but our eyes consist of an aperture (pupil), a lens (iris) and a photosensitive plate behind it called the retina. Light impacts the retina which sends a message via the optic nerves to the visual cortex at the back of our brain. The visual cortex interprets the light impinging upon the retina and tells us what we're seeing. This light is less than the image we're looking at, so our brain fills in the remainder of the image for us. So even the senses are governed by previous experience of what those particular patterns of light represent, rather than giving us a "pure" image, unadulterated by past experience.

Don't believe it?

Take the following expression:

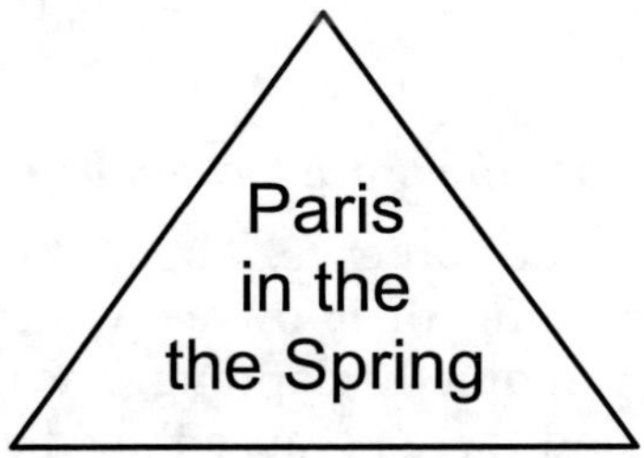

What does it say?

Write down the expression above on a piece of paper. O.K.....Does it say:

1. "Paris in the Spring"?

   or does it say

2. "Paris in the the Spring"?

Now take another look if you didn't see the extra "the". Isn't it amazing that you missed it!

Conditioning says there is one "the", sensory input says there are two. From now on you might be more cautious when you claim that you're right because you've seen it with your own eyes. What you've seen is what your brain tells you is there, not what actually *is* there. Perhaps what actually is there cannot be known because there's no uniformity of the apparatus of sight, no uniformity of experience and therefore no uniformity of interpretation. No wonder we're forever disagreeing with each other. The "known" and the "seen" are two very different things.

The following anecdote illustrates the difference between interpretations of reality

I was giving a talk at a conference on this very subject and I'd titled this talk:

"How what we* know *gets in the way of healing."

Another speaker, an international authority on health and well-being, introduced me. He looked at the title of my speech, hesitated a moment, and then said:

"Today we're very privileged to hear a talk from Dr Harrison titled:

"The more we know, the more we can heal ourselves."

I quickly looked at the audience. About ten people of the two hundred there, reading their own programs, were smiling eagerly. Some began quietly clapping. Those people could've walked out then and there because they'd already gotten the point.

I'm spending so much time on pre-conceived notions and what we think we already know because it's this same certainty that locks in our view of life, ourselves, and locks our healing capabilities into a diminished state of responsiveness.

And that provides us with a definition of illness.

Illness is a diminished responsiveness to internal and external imbalances which arise during the journey of life.

We need to be willing to risk our known view in order to heal.

And of course as soon as we take a risk we have to contend with the fear of the unknown.

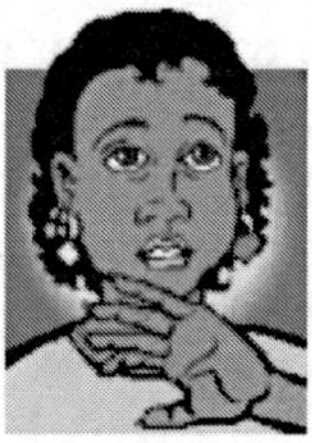

Many of us prefer the pain and suffering of the known to the fear of the unknown.

8
SECOND NATURE AND FIRST NATURE

Second Nature is what we've become, i.e. our attitudes, beliefs and opinions have become Second nature.

First Nature is what we were before the need to adapt to life.

The following diagram explains it.

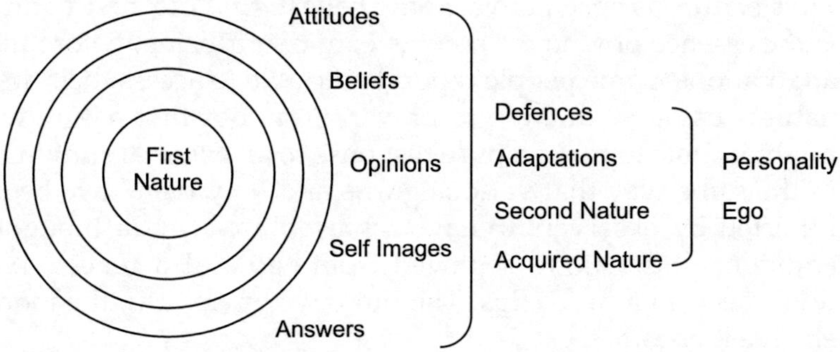

We acquire attitudes, beliefs, opinions, self-images and what we call "answers" as we progress through life. These are collectively called our defences or adaptations. They've become "second nature" and constitute our acquired nature. Another way of looking at these acquisitions is that they form our personality or our ego. First nature may be referred to as our "Self".

We respond to people and situations in our lives through the filters (blinkers, if you like) of our personality.

Our adaptations cocoon our first nature within a protective, defensive perimeter. We didn't acquire these defences for no reason. We acquired precisely the personality that we needed in order to survive. Some of our personality traits may have been initiated whilst we were in the womb and some perhaps even before that. The degree to which these traits are inherited and the degree to which they are acquired through life experience is unknown. Genetics is unfolding so quickly it's difficult to predict what will be known in the coming years. Nonetheless, pure sciences have a habit of being modified and at times contradicted by human experience. Perhaps this too is simply a lack of scientific advancement. Perhaps the random nature of the universe and the creatures in it will always defy both measurement and prediction. Uncertainty may be the fundamental architecture of our existence. Time may or may not tell.

Meanwhile we struggle to recover from illness as best we can, using whatever we have at our disposal.

First Nature is speculative. Some believe that our first nature is the essence of who we are, the core of our being, before the adaptations. Some people report being able to access their first natures using meditation or prayer. From our first nature we might be able to make a pure response to an external stimulus, in the same way that various gurus and holy men have been reported by observers to have achieved a clarity of thought, emotions and actions, removed from ego and defences. We don't need to aim for this. The more we grasp at it, the more elusive it becomes.

> ***The m3health Program loosens the grip of our second natures.***

Instead of a response dictated by past conditioning, we allow a different response, one that we don't consciously need to determine. We've all experienced this. Where once we would respond to a negative comment about us with anger, we may now be less affected by it. Take a simple example of a person who's shorter than most, and suffered the "short arse" taunts of children. After years of being frustrated and resentful because of it, and responding with anger whenever anyone mentioned it, he may mature beyond the taunt. Then, he's no longer affected by it.

He no longer criticises himself for being short and hence is unavailable for criticism from outsiders over being short.

For similar reasons, a person who likes his own blue eyes is completely unaffected by someone else criticising them.

Try this experiment.

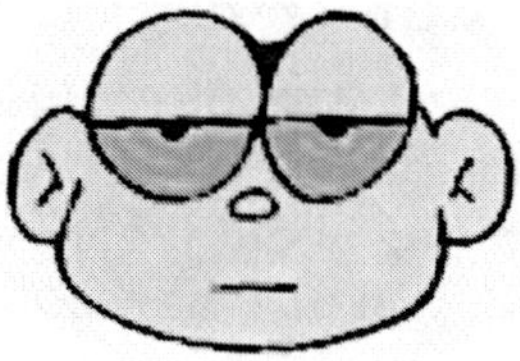

Ask a friend to criticise your eye colour. Eye colour is usually a good example as most people are happy enough with the colour of their eyes. If a person with blue eyes is criticised by another who likes brown eyes and not blue eyes, our blue eyed person responds with no response, indifference or perhaps faint amusement. Why doesn't the criticism touch him, even though on other matters he may be sensitive to criticism? Because he doesn't criticise himself for having blue eyes. Any criticism that hurts us is ultimately a criticism we make of ourselves, and someone else has simply recognised our self-criticism, perhaps recognising the impact it has, and wanting to hurt us. This can be simply demonstrated by asking someone to criticise you over a physical feature of yours that you don't like, and noting your response. Our own anger at ourselves (perhaps some of it guilt) is the source of much of our anger when we're criticised by another person.

And how exactly is an understanding of the origins of criticism of assistance in recovering from illness??

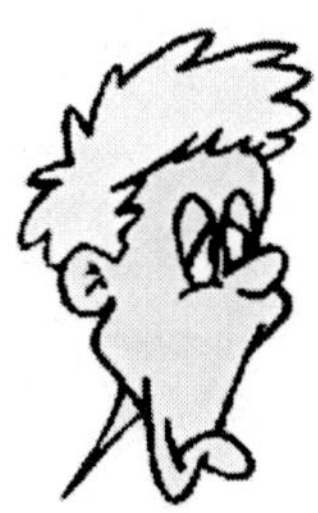

Underlying one's self criticism over any matter whether height, eye colour or any other more sophisticated criticism is the general self-criticism "there's something wrong with me—I'm not good enough". This belief was adopted under limited options as a child. Such a belief goes looking for justification, otherwise a schism develops between internal reality ("I'm not good enough") and external reality ("Life's a beach").

Illness is a very effective way of confirming a belief that we deserve to be suffering for not being good enough in some way. In the course of enquiring about the messages you received in your family as a child, you may have found that some of these self-critical messages surfaced. Just recognising that they aren't "true"—they're simply what your particular circumstances required you to adopt as the truth decommissions them. Time is required here as well as awareness.

Often we can't remember specific messages from parents that we weren't good enough, but our parents may well have demonstrated by their comments and actions that they felt inadequate and by implication, life was a place in which people feel inadequate. The child is obliged by inference to follow suit.

There may be a strong recurring pattern of illness running through families and whilst no doubt the inheritance of faulty genes or genetic mutations account for some of this, the factors we've been discussing are also significant, and perhaps more accessible.

Once again, we use whatever contributes to our recovery.

> ***To uncouple our lives and our immune systems from a belief that we weren't or aren't good enough, makes a great start to our recovery.***

An immune system that believes itself inadequate can't cure us.

9
IMMUNE SYSTEM

The way we think and feel about ourselves, others and life affects all our biological systems. We'll be aware of some of those effects, and others will be unknown to us.

This field is called psycho-neuro-immunology, a conglomerate term describing the three principle systems that are linked, namely the psychological, the nervous and the immune systems. Because science is moving so quickly in all fields, and none more so than in the biological sciences, today's research is often superseded or even in disrepute tomorrow. M3health is therefore loathe to justify any claims it may appear to be making using current scientific understanding, knowing that the justification will not last all that long. We prefer to invite people to use their intuition and their common sense instead of taking our assurances. Common sense is a complex understanding of the nature of things, some of which lies beyond reason and consciousness. Perhaps it has more to do with our "old brain" than our more recently acquired brain functions. Common sense needs to be allowed to have a say in what to explore, what's of value to us, how we can best survive and whether to continue with the m3health Program.

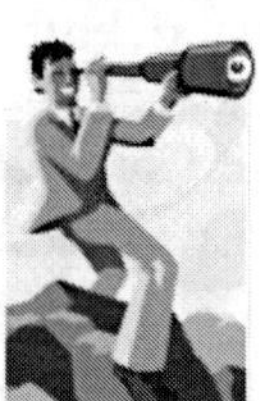

An inquiry, such as the m3health program, is open-ended. An open mind, employed in conjunction with whatever medications, surgery or counselling has been advised, is a powerful healer. If a person suffering from a serious or long-standing disease can let go of rigid thoughts and ideas, and at the same time begin to experience previously suppressed emotions, that person gives himself the best chance of recovery.

Exploring the very nature of belief, proof, validity, knowledge, answers, reality and certainty appear more helpful in recovering from illness than trying to validate the latest scientific theory.

However, for those of you who are unwilling to take any steps at all until there's some "proof" of the validity of the notion that our psychology profoundly affects our physical body, here's a snippet of contemporary science. Expect it to be substantially modified over the next few years. The synopsis is from the *British Medical Journal* in the year 2000. In addition further references are given.

"Many interactions occur between the immune, neural, and psychological systems. These interactions include communication pathways from the brain to the immune system, particularly the hypothalamic-pituitary-adrenal (HPA) axis and the autonomic nervous system, that mediate the influence of psychological variables, such as stress and emotions, on immunity and resistance to disease.

In addition, when the body is confronted by pathogens, the immune system serves as a sensory organ, alerting the brain to the presence of infection induced immune activation. The communication from the immune system to the brain is mediated by cytokines, which are peptides that orchestrate the immune response with a wide range of other biologic activities. During immune stimulation, cytokines such as interleukins and interferons are produced both in the periphery and in the brain, where they can affect neural, neuroendocrine, and behavioral functions through specific receptors."

- Ader R., Cohen N., Felten D. Psychoneuroimmunology: interactions between the nervous system and the immune system. *Lancet* 1995; 345: 99-103.
- Maier S.F., Watkins L.W. Implications of immune-to-brain communication for sickness and pain. *Proc. Natl. Acad. Sci.* USA 1999; 96: 7710-13.

- Dantzer R., Aubert A., Bluthe R.M., et al. Mechanisms of the effects of cytokines. In: Dantzer R., Wollman E.E., Yirmiya R., eds. *Cytokines, Stress and Depression*. New York: Kluwer Academic/Plenum Publishers; 1999: 83-106.

  Kenneth V. lserson [West J. Med. 173(5):333-36, 2000. © 2000 BMJ, Inc.]

- Lipton, Bruce. The Biology of Belief 2005.

10
THOUGHTS

"I can't help what I

think....

I'm being thunk!!"

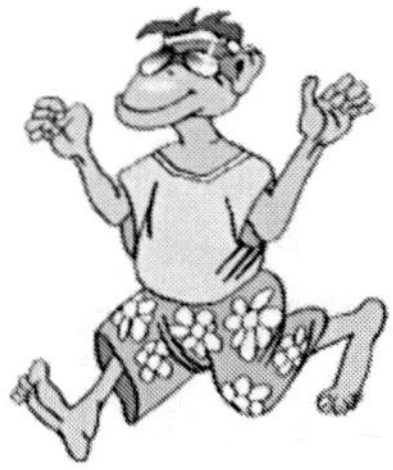

Responses to stimuli include actions, thoughts and feelings. These three components of a response often occur simultaneously and the boundaries defining them are blurred. For example a thought could be regarded as a complex set of feelings represented by a sequence of words. An emotion could be described as the biochemical representation of a thought, or the physiological response to a thought. Actions may be automatic reactions to thoughts and feelings.

Thoughts are our response to a stimulus from outside of ourselves or from a bodily sensation. In either case we don't consciously choose the circumstances that initiated the thought, and in that sense our thought is an automatic response, not an intentional creation of ours.

A thought provoking way of expressing this might be to say that....

"We can't help what we think."

Since factors outside of our consciousness are initiating our thoughts, one way of looking at this is to say that...

"the Universe is 'thinking us'"

Both our external and internal environment are part of that Universe.

We're a biological organism responding to a stimulus with a thought. Another way of saying this is that......

"we're being thunk!"

This is the opposite of a popular approach by many new age authors who believe that you can create your own reality by choosing to think certain thoughts. Repetition of the "good" thoughts then causes a change in the reality.

It is the contention of m3health that the content of the thoughts is irrelevant. It matters not whether someone categorizes them as "good" or "bad". The rigidity with which they're held leads to a rigid immune response. The realisation that "negative" thoughts need addressing however, raises awareness, and serves an important function.

Whilst some of us might agree that "We can't help what someone else thinks", we might find it more difficult to take the next step which explores the notion that "I can't help what I think." This recognises that a thought is an outcome of a meeting between our current situation and our past conditioning, neither of which is...or was...under our control.

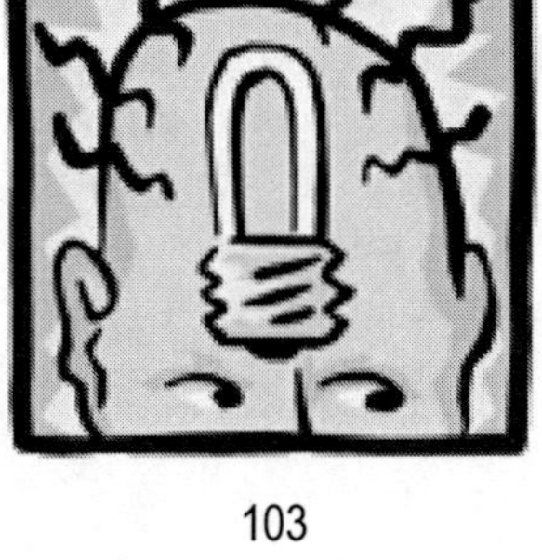

We're often a prisoner of our own thoughts.

We treat our thoughts as if they're reality. We believe them. Whilst it's indeed us who gives them expression, we haven't created them consciously. They're an automatic response. They seem real, but they may not be "reality". It's us who assigns reality to them.

> ***Imagine what it would be like to not believe what you think any more than you believe what someone else thinks!***

All of this starts to get tricky of course, and we don't claim to know exactly how humans think, or who the entity is, who's doing the thinking. It's clear however, that most of the time most of us are relating to our thought processes as if they represent universal truths or universal reality when a cursory examination of them indicates that this is far from the case.

We regard what we think as the truth since this makes life easy by eliminating the need to consider a whole range of equally plausible "truths". Another reason we're inclined to believe our own thoughts is that we don't have to modify our thoughts for any other human being. There need be no saving face, no politeness, no politics in a thought, since no-one else is privy to it. But this lack of adaptation to suit others doesn't make it the truth either.

The notion that our thoughts aren't true is so alien to most people that they have trouble grasping it. We believe what we think so implicitly that we don't even recognise our beliefs as no more than thoughts. We behave as if the thought and us are the same thing. We make no distinction between ourselves and our thoughts. We believe what we hear ourselves say. Imagine not operating like this. Imagine becoming aware of a thought stream running through our heads and becoming an impartial observer, simply watching it. The question of whether the thoughts are true or not never arises. We don't question if a cold, rainy morning is "true" any more than we question the truth of a warm, sunny morning. The notion is ridiculous. We control neither morning. Introducing a distinction between the thoughts and ourselves is a major step in stopping our thoughts from "running us".

Our thoughts are responses that our set of adaptations and defences—our conditioning—guarantee. Anyone else who'd been through our particular background, and found herself in our current circumstances, would presumably be having the same thoughts. (I say "presumably" because of course I wouldn't really know—the idea is to explore the notion, not insist upon its veracity). Given the stimulus, our thoughts are guaranteed by our second natures or personalities. If we allow the thoughts to continue to be treated as though they are us, our lives and our physiologies will also be run by the past, unable to respond freely in the present, and unable to effectively respond to the threat of either a loss, or an invasion. With a compromised immune system, illness is made more likely.

If we can begin to recognise the entity who's experiencing the thoughts rather than regarding ourselves and our thoughts as inseparable, we can begin the process of decommissioning the power exercised over many of us by our thoughts. To recap some of the thoughts which cause us so much trouble, "I'm not good enough", "I'm stupid", "No-one can help me", "Everyone's a schmuck", "I'm stupid", "I'm never going to be free of this illness" etc.........etc......

Or those which alienate us from our peers.... "People are hopeless"...."Why can't anyone understand me".... "Why is it always me".... "No-one can ever help me".... "Nothing ever seems to work".... "This is all a load of crap"......etc...etc....

Then there are the thoughts that are regarded by many people as conducive to health such as "I'm a really lovely person", "life is what you make it", "people make their own luck", or "I care for myself more and more each day". As mentioned previously, the actual thoughts are irrelevant. What matters is the conviction with which they're held for this is the same energy, and the same degree, to which they reduce the effectiveness of our own healing systems.

It might be helpful to write down some of the thoughts that you can now see are running your life.

They're often related to the following commonly contentious areas of our lives.

Personal capabilities

Work performance

Achievements

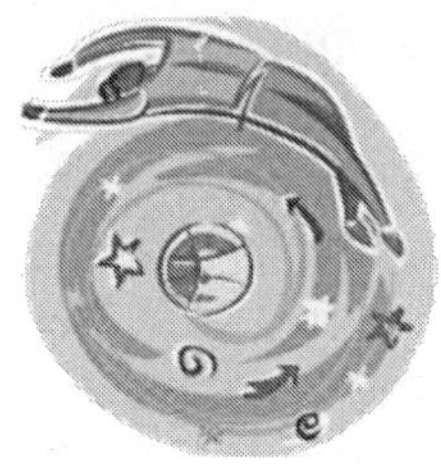

Sexuality

Gender

Parenting

Childhood

Hardly done by

Physical appearance

Thoughts are so important to us in the m3health journey that we must return to them time and again.

The following process may provide an experience of the separateness of thought and thinker.

Allow yourself to be quiet for a while, perhaps sitting or lying comfortably and just becoming aware of your breathing. You may be aware that as you breathe your abdomen rises and falls, or you may notice the sensation of the air moving past your nostrils. By concentrating on the breathing, thoughts may be temporarily suspended.

As soon as you have a thought, any thought (which will happen almost immediately), note what the thought is. It could be anything from "This is silly".... "This is bizarre"... to "Wow, this is interesting", or "My foot aches". Note the thought. There's no need to say or do anything. Noting the thought means simply acknowledging it. Go back to watching your breathing, noting your abdomen rise and fall with your breath, or becoming aware of the air flowing through your nostrils, and await the next thought. You don't know what it will be. You aren't creating it. You're sitting and waiting for it to arrive. You can be sure that it won't take long.

You're waiting for the Universe to think using the agency of one of its organisms...you. Had anyone else been in your shoes they'd be having the same thoughts. The thoughts are an interaction between your past experience and a present time stimulus.

What have your thoughts got to do with you personally?

Not much.

Can you see that using this model there's no point trying to change your "negative" thoughts into "positive" thoughts.

A. "Negative" and "Positive" are artificial classifications. Both are criticisms in the sense that both are judgements.

B. They aren't yours to change anyway.

C. The thoughts are a response of your past, which you didn't create, to present circumstances that you didn't create either. To try and change your thoughts is to try and change two factors over which you have no power and no control.

D. Your thoughts are decommissioned from doing you further damage by recognising that they aren't you and they aren't reality.

The content of your thoughts becomes irrelevant, and hence you welcome any thoughts that might come your way. In the healthiest individuals thoughts enter and leave without interruption. They are not assigned importance or meaning.

Like an empty vessel or musical instrument....

The thinker becomes a hollow bamboo, vibrating in harmony with her surroundings as thoughts flow unimpeded through her being.

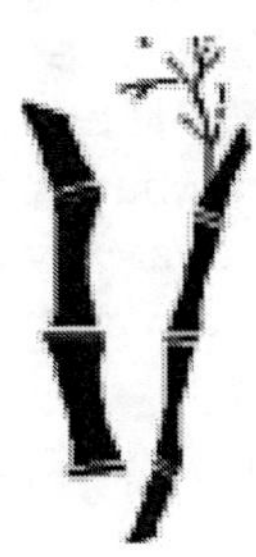

11
FEELINGS

Feelings or emotions constitute another of the powerful human responses.

The four basic feelings are anger, sadness, fear and joy. It helps at the outset of this chapter to get in touch with each of these, acting them out so as to re-familiarise yourself with what they are, and what sensations accompany them. Let's do that now.

Anger Shake your fists and shout Grrrrrrrrr..........

Sadness Try and conjure up a sad image and see if you can cry.

Fear Imagine you're being attacked. Shake and tremble and look frightened.

Joy Jump in the air shouting Wheeeee...............

Silly.... I know...... but it might get you in the mood, for many of us have suppressed some or even all of our emotions and are now unable to feel them or even recognise that we're feeling them. Repressing emotions may have a serious impact on the nervous system and the immune system. I'm using the terms "feelings" and "emotions" interchangeably in the m3health Program.

What are emotions?

They are physiological mechanisms that rejuvenate and energise the body and mind. They are a discharge of tension and a release of energy. They enable us to re-establish equilibrium after an event that could be a danger to us, or an event that has initiated a physiological response within us. Emotions can be protective, by warning an assailant not to mess with us by a display of anger for example, or can invite empathy such as in crying or can bring people closer together as in a group display of joy and celebration. Because emotions are a collision between the present and the past, they have significant evolutionary functions to perform, navigating complex social and environmental situations.

Emotions can be complex. They often co-exist, or occur in sequence. It's difficult to conceive of circumstances in which anger can exist alone, for example. It appears to be always preceded by fear. Anger at the threat of losing a loved one or at being assaulted is not the same as anger expressed when you hit your thumb with a hammer. This latter may not be anger at all in its pure form but rather an exclamation of pain that has the physical appearance of anger. Or it may derive from the thought "I'm an idiot", giving rise to a feeling of hopelessness and inadequacy, themselves pre-cursors to the fear of not being sufficiently lovable to be able to stay safe and stay alive.

Guilt, one of the most common emotions, happens when an individual is angry with himself, often for harming another, but it may be more complex than that. We can be angry with things, with other people or angry with ourselves.

Feeling responsible is another complex emotion, not quite the same as guilt perhaps, but containing elements of anger, sadness and perhaps fear. We can feel multiple emotions at the same time, such as when a loved one who's been suffering finally dies, causing us to feel both great sadness and great relief — "mixed feelings" we often say. Feeling loss, (fear and sadness) uncomfortable, (fear with physiological discomfort), anxious, (fear) frustrated, (anger), regret, (sadness and guilt), hopeless, etc. are combinations or variations of the common feeling states. There are, of course, many more than listed here.

It isn't necessary to go through the exercise of trying to work out exactly what it is that we're feeling, and where it comes from, it will at best anyway be an approximation, but it may be important to allow whatever feelings are trying to arise to do so.

Many of us express one feeling in order to mask or repress another feeling that's more problematic for us. Men may express anger when they're feeling sad or frightened or even tender. Women may cry when they're feeling angry or scared. There are also cultural and religious variations in the expression of emotions. It's commonly accepted (and therefore not necessarily true ☺) that the Latin races are often quicker to express anger than the Anglo Saxons, who prefer not to express emotions at all, but rather try and think themselves through situations. In this case rather than replace one emotion with another, the whole raft of emotions is replaced by thinking. Such generalisations across cultures are interesting but perhaps of not much importance to the individual trying to recover from illness or prevent illness by maintaining a healthy set of emotional responses.

The following questions help us to learn more about our own method of expressing or repressing emotions.

- When was the last time you expressed anger?
- What did you call it? (Pissed, peeved, annoyed, irritated, bothered, frustrated, furious, disrespected, irate.....)
- Are you prepared to acknowledge it for what it was, or do you prefer to explain it away, such as in the phrase "I wasn't reeeeaaaaally feeling angry".
- Did you explain it away?

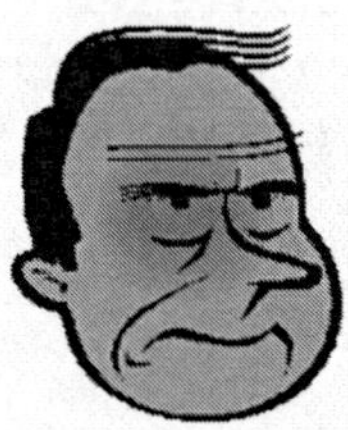

- Why did you stop expressing anger and start thinking instead?
- On reflection, was there more anger to come when you decided to stop?
- Are you irritated much of the time?
- With what are you angry?
- With whom are you angry?
- When was the first time in your life you can recall being angry?

- Did your father express anger?
- Did your mother express anger?
- What was said about anger in your family?
- What are your beliefs about the safety of expressing anger?

ANGER AND SOCIETY

Society is very frightened of anger. Social institutions and governments are very concerned with any expression of dissent, and so it's no surprise that academics and clinicians who research anger publish papers which demonstrate unequivocally that the expression of anger is........ and here comes their favoured term .... dangerous! All scientific research is influenced at some level by social forces dictating its outcome even if not recognised by the researchers.

In the case of anger, differentiation is rarely made between the natural spontaneous expression of anger, and acting upon anger that's directed towards another individual. Yet they are quite different.

If anger has another person or our self as its object, it's not the sort of anger that heals, but an expression of violence.

Violence is anger with an object.

Hence much research reveals that men who are violent towards other people continue to be violent, and concludes therefore that the expression of anger leaves the person expressing it feeling worse off, and with serious consequences for the object of his anger, and for himself.

The anger cycle is reinforced by violence.

On the other hand, a healthy yell dissipates anger rather than reinforces it. In the expression of healthy anger there's no thought directing the emotion towards any object or person. There's no thoughts at all. There's no object of the anger since the emotion has been triggered by an event and the individual has reacted spontaneously, without thinking, i.e. without having thoughts.

Anger heals when it has no object.

Anger that has an object harms, irrespective of whether the object of our anger is us, an object, or someone else.

SADNESS

Men commonly repress anger. Few men cry freely. It feels wonderful to have a good cry, but social restraints upon men in most Western societies forbid men to cry even if crying promotes health. This remains the case until a chronic disease that won't seem to shift using conventional therapies comes along. When the discomfort of the dis-ease exceeds the fear of appearing unmanly, the sufferer may risk a few tears. Gradually he may become accustomed to crying and feels much better for it. Let's take a look at your own sadness.

- Do you cry freely?
- When was the last time you had a "good cry"?
- What did that feel like?
- Can you recall crying as a child?

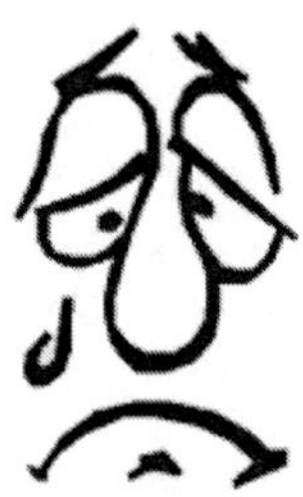

- Did anyone inform you that crying was not a good thing to do? (Men may recall the prohibition of "Boys don't cry!")
- Do you suffer from chronic sinusitis, recurrent eye infections, rhinitis or chronic repeated sore throats?
- Are your eyes often irritated or itchy?
- Do you suffer from the flu more than most?

These are some of the common complaints amongst the non-crying group of men commonly seen in a general medical practice.

JOY

Joy is possibly more suppressed in contemporary society than any other emotion.

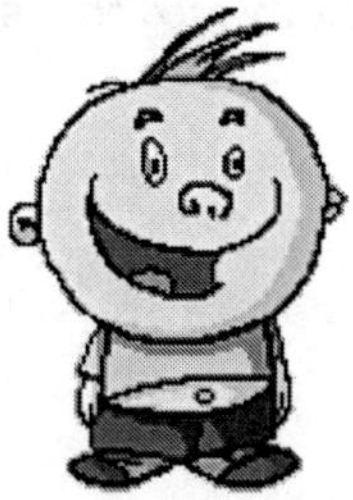

Many of us have no permission to be joyful, for wherever we look we see someone who's suffering, and it seems callous to express joy in those circumstances. As a consequence we hold joy in and only permit ourselves a wry smile when it would be healthier to be jumping in the air with glee. Children mercifully have more permission to express joy, at least for a while until they start to annoy the grownups. Laughing is biologically complex and has been attributed with all manner of medical benefits. To discover whether we've been suppressing joy the following questions may help.

- Do you allow yourself to express unbridled joy?
- When was the last time you really let yourself go and had a good laugh?
- What tends to stop you expressing joy?
- Are there any admonishments in your mind when you try and enjoy yourself?
- Have you considered the word "en-joy" before? It means to put joy into.
- Do you find yourself stopping your kids from expressing joy or other emotions they may be feeling?
- Do you get annoyed with the noisy laughter of children?

- Was there anyone living with you as a child who was sad or upset much of the time?
- Were you frequently instructed by a parent to tone down your zest for life, your vibrancy, your humour, your laughter?
- Can you remember the saying "Children should be seen and not heard"? (or was that just from my generation?)
- Do you feel that being joyful is silly or immature, or of little value?
- Are you critical of others who are openly enjoying themselves?
- What have you been putting off which you'd love to do?

FEAR

Fear is the least recognised of the feeling states because it's often low grade and we become so accustomed to it that we fail to recognise it. We have other names for it. We say that we're anxious, nervous, apprehensive or insecure. These are all synonyms for fear.

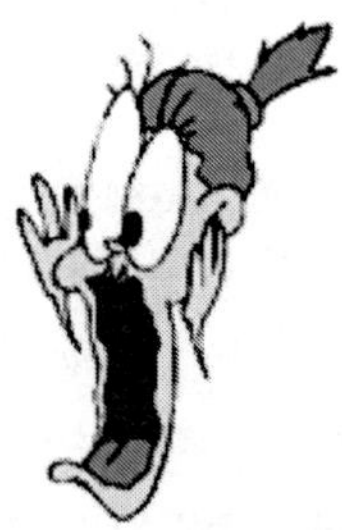

We can recognise fear by the powerful physiological changes it causes. "Fight or flight" is a long-standing way of expressing the actions we may take if we feel fear or anger. Both responses result in raised blood pressure, dilated pupils, increased heart rate, sweating and a re-distribution of blood to those systems we need in a hurry. With such major physiological effects it's not surprising that consequences may accrue from their lack of expression. Fear appears to underlie all anger, for if there were no threat to the organism, there'd be no point in becoming angry. Anger is the response of an organism under attack, and feeling fear. A function of the anger is to look fierce and to cause an aggressor to think twice about attacking.

When things change, we feel fear.

The change may be minor, such as a road closed unexpectedly on the drive to work. And the fear may be correspondingly minor so that all we register is an irritation, a minor state of anger covering the fear of being late for work. A significant change in our lives will always be accompanied by some fear, expressed or repressed. When one looks at a list of events in people's lives which cause most anxiety, the large changes such as house moving or renovations, getting married, the death of a loved one and loss of a job are at the top of the list. There are as many "good" things at the top of the list as there are "bad" things – it's the change itself that creates the anxiety. Many people report that the onset of an illness coincides with such times. Our own relationship with fear is often heavily masked.

The following questions may help you to recognise if you're trying to avoid experiencing the emotion of fear. Most of us do this by trying, sometimes desperately, to control life.

The same controls we use to protect us against the unknown, are also applied to our immune system, limiting its response.

- When did you last feel fear?
- What did it feel like?
- Do you seek circumstances in which fear is prevalent, such as terrifying rides at amusement parks, extreme sports or driving recklessly?

Fear attached to joy is called excitement. The rush of adrenalin combined with the semi-controlled nature of the experience is much sought after by many people.

- Are you suffering from anxiety?
- Would you call yourself an anxious person?
- Are you capable of shaking and trembling with fear?
- Do you become very still when you're afraid?
- Are you the person who "keeps it together" when all around you have "lost it"?

- Are you heavily relied upon by family and friends when the going gets tough?
- Are you the person nobody needs to take care of because you always manage?
- Do you like watching scary movies?
- Do you have nightmares?
- Do you like things to be ordered?
- Are you the person who insists upon everything conforming to the rules?
- When was the last time you broke the law knowingly?
- How do you relate to those in authority?
- Are you a creature of habit?
- Are you always on time?
- What's your explanation for that?
- Does your children's untidiness bother you?
- How many jobs have you had in your life?
- How many career changes have you had?
- Do you like working for large organisations?
- Do you prefer working for yourself?
- Are your vacations always planned in advance?
- Do you ever just "take off", not knowing where you're going or how you're going to get there?
- Is your life "air conditioned"?
- Do you try and "sanitise" situations?
- What are the most important things for you in your life?
- Which people are most important?
- What could you least do without in your life?
- What causes you most distress?
- Do you regard yourself as anxious?
- In what circumstances do you feel anxiety most acutely?

- Have you felt the need to inform anyone that you're undertaking this m3health Program?
- Who would you like to inform but have not done so to date?
- What prevents you from discussing it with others?
- Do you maintain a calm exterior whilst underneath you feel anxious?
- What do you understand by the phrase, "the need to stay in control"?
- Are you a controlling person?
- Are you working in an organisation that's responsible for controlling a group of people?
- Do you hold strong views about other people's behaviour?
- Do you have a legal qualification?
- Do you have a psychiatric/psychological/social work qualification?
- Are you a politician?
- Are you a member of the Police Force or the Armed Services?
- Are you a member of any body or organisation with a statutory power to judge others?
- Do you feel safer when you have the backing of a large organisation?
- Are you a career public servant?
- Do you think you know what's best for others?
- Are you a very ordered person?
- Do you like to get your own way?
- Are you a "know all"?
- Do other people defer to your superior knowledge?
- Are you better prepared with briefs than others whom you know?

- Did you study a lot as a child?
- Are you forever studying new information?
- Are you a cross word fanatic?
- Do you find yourself interrupting people?
- Do you interrupt a conversation when you want to say something?
- Would you say that you ... "don't suffer fools gladly!"?
- What would be the most offensive thing that someone could say of you?
- Are you always arranging circumstances to suit yourself?
- Do you find it uncomfortable "just going along for the ride"?
- Do you always like to know what's going on?
- Do you find yourself keeping tabs on loved ones, friends and associates?
- Are you a firm believer in the dictum that "If you want it done well, you must do it yourself"?
- Do you find it hard delegating authority?
- When was the last time you did something spontaneous?
- Do you do things that are perhaps a little mad?
- Are you enjoying going through this series of questions?
- Do they irritate you?
- Are you often irritated?
- Are you generally annoyed with children?
- How much time do you, or did you spend with your own children?
- Did you consciously choose not to have children in your life?
- Why was that?
- When was that?
- In retrospect do you still feel the same?

- Are you a nervous traveller when someone else is driving?
- Are you a creature of habit?

We've spent some time looking at fear because of its pivotal role in our m3health Program. The need to live within the "known" can be a powerful disincentive to take the risks required for recovery. As Krishnamurti implies in the title of his work *Freedom from the Known,* freedom may be the reward for being prepared to forgo the known. However, to do so will require the willingness, however slowly, to experience the fear of the unknown.

What's so uncomfortable about fear?

Is it the bodily sensations?

Is it the mental anguish?

If fear were genuinely terrible, how to explain why people are so attracted to fear and why so many of our recreational activities from roller coasters to skydiving are designed to experience it. In these circumstances people love being afraid—they're "up for it". They like it. They like the adrenalin and the endomorphins that are released, giving them a natural "high". This sort of fear seems different from the fear we experience if we transgress old taboos. And therein may lie the difference.

> ***The old fear left over from childhood, when we feared not being able to survive, and resulted in us adopting a protective "second nature", is the fear we don't like.***

We don't like re-experiencing the old fear, perhaps best expressed as the *fear of the fear*.

As children we were helpless and couldn't keep ourselves alive. We had little option but to toe the parental line, resulting in frequent anxiety.

If the expression of fear and dissent wasn't tolerated as a child, we tend to bottle and suppress the emotions now. The child may have registered bucking the system as life threatening. Mostly we were unable to prosecute our needs due to our physical size, and every time we try and assert our independence and freedom as a grown up, we may re-experience old leftover fears.

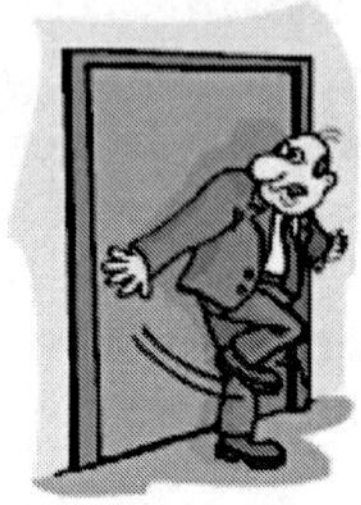

Of course the fear isn't life threatening now, since we now keep ourselves alive, and probably wasn't then, but we didn't know that. Fear may remain powerful enough as an adult to immobilise us, and have us retreat into known methods of managing it, which is, to suppress it.

Anxiety is the result of suppressing fear.

12
EMOTIONS... EXPRESS OR REPRESS

Emotional starvation

Emotional Health

Emotional Obesity

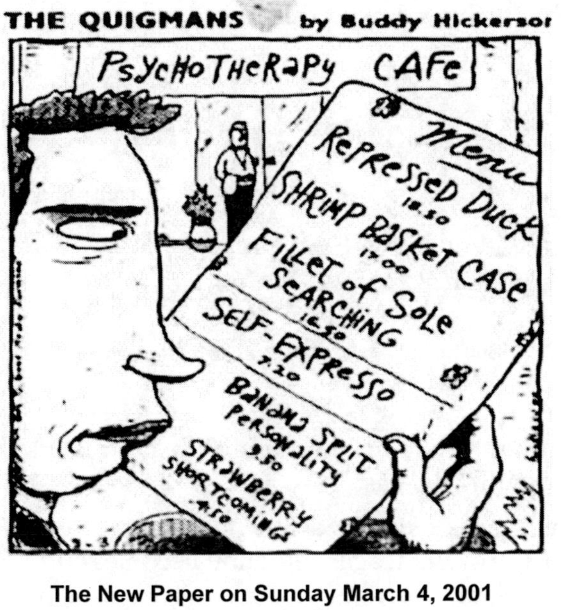
THE QUIGMANS by Buddy Hickerson
PSYCHOTHERAPY CAFE
Menu
REPRESSED DUCK 10.50
SHRIMP BASKET CASE 17.00
FILLET OF SOLE SEARCHING 16.50
SELF-EXPRESSO 7.20
BANANA SPLIT PERSONALITY 9.50
STRAWBERRY SHORTCOMINGS 4.50

The New Paper on Sunday March 4, 2001

Emotions, like all other physiological systems, need exercise for health. Under-use and over-use both cause problems eventually.

We're familiar with the term emotional starvation and emotional health but less familiar perhaps with emotional obesity. Taking a look at eating patterns helps to understand this.

When we haven't eaten our lowered blood sugar level causes hunger so that we eat. When the blood sugar level rises we stop eating because we're no longer hungry. If we continue to eat we raise our blood sugar levels excessively and obesity results.

In a similar way the exercise of emotions can be healthy for the system or unhealthy, depending on the degree to which the expression is natural. Expressing emotions from first nature is more natural than from second nature, where they are more contaminated.

The following diagram shows the consequences of expressing or repressing emotions.

A graph further down this section explains the levels mentioned.

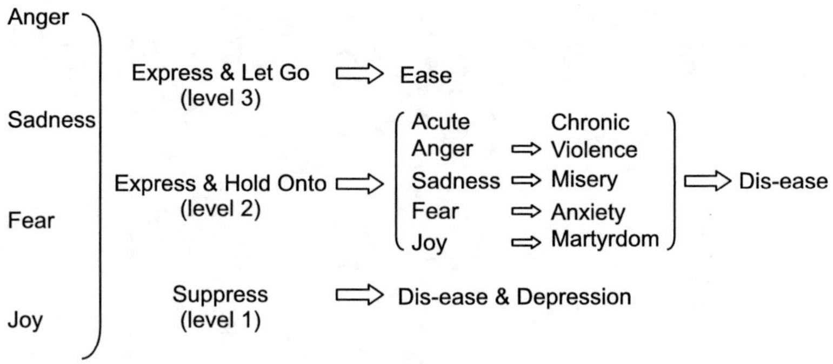

Expressing an emotion, then letting it go, results in "ease", compared with "dis-ease".

If the emotion is expressed but not allowed to finish, i.e. is held onto, the original acute emotion becomes chronic. Instead of the organism returning to a resting level of physiological activity, the emotional energy remains un-discharged and creates emotional tension within the organism. This may not matter in the short-term but over a longer period, repeated emotional repression is followed by physiological change and then anatomical change. This is called pathology.

Each separate acute emotion, if held onto, results in a different chronic feeling. Unreleased anger leads to someone being described as an "angry old bugger", or if a younger man, a "violent young man". Women, increasingly freed from the social restraints which shackled their mothers, are also acting out more of their internal anger and becoming violent. Chronic sadness in an individual results in a miserable person unable to see any good anywhere, whereas chronic fear results in anxiety often with intermittent panic.

Unreleased joy I've termed "martyrdom", but that isn't quite correct. I'd like someone to write and tell me what he thinks the fixed smile and "mustn't grumble" attitude of the person intent on not releasing joy might be better termed.

The chronic feeling states are maintained for safety. Rather than experience an acute emotion that was forbidden as a child, those feelings that are more acceptable to parents and to cultures, are allowed. Hence the angry old man might really be feeling sorrow, but fifty years on from the original admonishments not to cry, he's still uncomfortable with sadness and simply replaces it and other emotions with anger, which results in him feeling aggrieved much of the time.

Why would anyone hold onto a parental directive fifty years later? Everyone in this field has their own view on this, so don't take mine as being any "truer" than your own or someone else's. I try and run explanations past a "common sense" detector. They will change over time, but here's one way of looking at it.

The adult keeps fulfilling parental and societal messages because he adopted them under a set of very compromised conditions, i.e. he couldn't keep himself alive. He was totally helpless as a small baby unable to fulfil even his basic needs and consequently was very susceptible to external influences.

He acquired his preferred way of seeing and feeling things in those days, they became "second nature" to him, and he built his self-esteem around them. Then he built his "community" around them, congregating for safety with like-minded individuals. Every time he tries to throw off the shackles of early childhood conditioning, he experiences the same fear that resulted in him acquiring the adaptations or defences in the first place.

But he no longer needs anyone to keep him alive, I hear you protesting. True. But the old circuitry is still there, the parent in his head if you like, and now, as an adult, he risks being disapproved of by himself if he transgresses those early directives. In the intervening years he's built his own circle of family, friends and acquaintances on the foundations of the childhood defences, and he risks being censured by his tribe if he changes anything, particularly his partner who chose him specifically because of his personality.

The risk in doing anything different is the loss of love or belonging.

When the suffering of the current circumstances exceeds the fear of doing, feeling and thinking something different, we consider alternatives, one of which might be to undertake the m3health Program. There are other circumstances in which people grow and change other than suffering, but disease which is not responding to conventional therapy is a common reason people give for taking a risk.

If emotions are suppressed completely, the person feels nothing.

Depression is the consequence and disease often follows.

Depression has been regarded as chronic sadness, but I prefer the explanation that an absence of feelings is more akin to depression. Much is known about the biochemistry of depression and many drugs are on the market for remedying the underlying chemical imbalances. As with all of medicine, it's up to the individual to decide how much his depression is a consequence of early childhood messages which he hasn't yet dealt with, and how much is a genetically inherited trait resulting in a biochemical imbalance to which no amount of self-reflection will make any difference.

Medication may be effective in alleviating the symptoms of the depression but will often not assist in the Inquiry. Most people suffering from depression have multiple episodes from which they recover and often some different medication is required as the disease continues. Many have also tried "talking therapy" often with a counsellor, psychologist or psychiatrist. This can be very helpful. Physical exercise is probably as valuable an "external" prescription as anything, but difficult to undertake when you're feeling totally flat.

The psychiatrist's need to be dispensing drugs, and the talking therapist's personal bias, both have to be taken into account by the patient in assessing whose needs are primarily being met by his treatment.

The following graph demonstrates the rise and fall of the emotions.

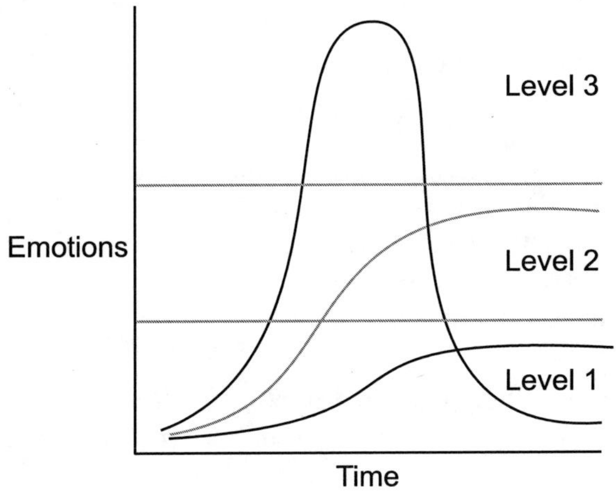

The highest curve indicates an emotion which arises, is expressed and disappears, leaving no residual physiological imbalance. The middle curve represents an emotion that arises and is held onto.

It may gradually fall away over time. The lowest curve is an emotion which remains sub-acute (not expressed at all) and is not recognised by the individual. The area under the lower two graphs indicates the residual emotions which alter physiology and eventually cause disease. They represent residual physiological imbalance.

Let's take a look at emotions we resist allowing to complete themselves, commonly felt feelings, and feelings that we never seem to get in touch with.

Here are some questions to assist.

- Do you believe that your disease has anything to do with your emotions?
- Do you prefer the nature (genetically inherited) or nurture (early childhood conditioning) explanation of emotional difficulties?
- Do you believe that your emotions can affect your state of physical health?

In answering these sorts of questions we have a valuable opportunity to listen to the voice in our heads..... called our thoughts. Remember the notion of "being thunk" and of introducing the third party—the listener—to the conversation between a biological organism, you, and the universe which spawned it. The Universe is here represented by the questions. The thoughts arise when the biological organism responds to the questions. The third party is neither creating the questions nor making the responses. He is a listener. An observer who only listens and watches.

By introducing a third party, the "listener", you need no longer identify with your thoughts.

The more independent you are from your thoughts, the more independence you give your immune system. An independent immune system is free to align itself with our "First Nature", before we modified it and controlled it in order to survive, turning it into "Second Nature".

First nature strives to be re-connected to the source of energy and of life. This is nature.

- What emotions do you most commonly feel?
- What emotions do you rarely or never feel?
- Which emotions in others create most discomfort for you?
- Would you like to explore experiencing the emotions that you find difficult?

13
ANGER

Anger is one emotion it's easy to get angry discussing. Fear is another. Let's take a look at anger specifically so that we might better recognise it and utilise it. Here are some general principles.

ANGER IS HEALTHY

Anger, along with the other emotions, is a conduit between the soma and the psyche, the body and the mind. Thoughts also link the physical and mental but perhaps not so obviously since thoughts appear to have no direct physiological consequences. The effect of thoughts may be mediated by the emotions that they generate and with which they're associated. For example the thought, "I'll never recover from this illness" may have no physical ramifications per se, but creates problems through its association with the affiliated feelings of helplessness and hopelessness, themselves descriptions of a hybrid of fear and sadness. As mentioned previously, the thought content is irrelevant. If the associated feelings were allowed full expression there would also be no consequences.

Disease is a consequence of unfinished physiological responses.

We have made much before of the need to keep all physiological systems in the body active to prevent the development of habitual pathways of repression, that lead to disturbed physiology and eventually pathology. Exercising the emotions, like exercising the body, is true preventative medicine. We will consider the differences between prevention and early detection later.

OWN YOUR OWN ANGER

Whilst most of us get angry with similar things such as a partner abandoning us or a motorist cutting in front of us on the road, the degree and specificity of our anger is unique to us. This is because much of what we recognise as anger is anger with a focus—another person, or an object (blame) or anger directed towards our self (guilt). Natural anger arising for example, from a denial of love or a denial of food is common to all humans and perhaps other species. Anger with an object is a response to our earlier conditioning and a defence mechanism. The expression of anger differs from one person to the next because we all had different upbringings. Anger with an object is part of an individual's personality.

"YOU MAKE ME ANGRY!"

We claim that other people and events make us angry, but the more likely explanation is that we're already angry and the event simply triggered and unmasked the old anger. The event didn't "make" us angry. By claiming that someone else is responsible for us feeling angry we deny it as our own, and by implication, that we can do anything about it. However, our claim that something "makes us angry" provides the opportunity for a closer look at a vital energy which we might harness for our own good, rather than it remain a hidden and denied factor in our disease. We may finally get into a relationship with our own anger in which we find ourselves saying to someone who's "made us angry"........*"Boy, I really got in touch with anger over what you did. I appreciate the opportunity of sorting this one out."* (Sounds farcical at first glance, doesn't it. Try saying it quietly to yourself.)

I'M NEVER ANGRY AT WHAT I SAY I AM

We all recognise that others get angry about minor matters when they're really upset about something else. We may even recognise it in ourselves, mostly a while after the event. If we aren't really angry at what we say we are, then what are we angry about?

To explore this we need to return to the first times in our lives when we experienced anger, before the defences were acquired. The child gets angry at either a loss or an invasion. The loss is withdrawal of whatever keeps him alive, which is food and love. The fear of invasion occurs whenever he's physically threatened. Animals in the wild, who appear not to acquire second natures but retain their first natures, still exhibit "anger" under those same circumstances. We probably do the same, though socialisation and our conditioning forces us to deny it, and to attach the anger to some other cause.

It's been suggested that fear underlies all anger. The child has the response of anger because he's afraid that if he doesn't get what he wants he cannot keep himself alive. The same fears remain in the adult, but now it isn't loss of food, but loss of approval, or love. The withdrawal of love by parents is no longer life threatening, but our partners, families and perhaps more importantly, our tribe or community take their place. The withdrawal of their approval may not be life threatening in the same sense as denial of food to the baby, but cast out from their community, people wither and die.

Being prepared to address the question "*with whom or with what am I really angry?*" is vital to healing. Let's proceed with it now.

Take your time with the following questions.

- What **makes** you angry?

  Make a list of all the things that really annoy you. Then narrow down the list until you have only a few left.
- Can you recall the last few times when you experienced anger?
- Recall what they were about.
- Who really annoys you?
- What is it about them that annoys you?
- Is there some recurring annoyance in your life which has been attached to various people and things over the years but which you recognise as familiar?
- As a child, did you experience anger towards anyone?
- What was your position in your family?

- Was there a sibling born when you were less than two years of age?
- Was there a brother or sister who was a favourite of either of your parents?
- Were you brought up by people who weren't your biological parents?
- Did your parents stay together when you were a child?
- If one parent left the marriage how old were you when that happened?
- Do women really annoy you?
- Do men really annoy you?
- Was there a bereavement in your family when you were a young child?
- Did you have to go into hospital below the age of 2 years for a period exceeding a week?

(This question will be difficult to answer without asking others.)

Did either parent leave home for any reason for two weeks when you were less than 2 years old?

The reason for these questions is that a small child registers the absence of a parent, particularly the prime caregiver, as an abandonment if the absence is more than about a week and if the child is below two years of age. These are far from fixed or reliable figures. Probably more important is the implication that a parent could leave or withdraw love or support. The child, powerless to do anything about this, lives in a constant state of anxiety. As a grown up, a potential loss of love, esteem, recognition or approval by loved ones, the peer group, the boss at work or the community, could initiate the old anxiety...... leading to fury.

What have you discovered about your own anger?

- Would you regard yourself as habitually angry?
- What emotion might be being masked by your anger?
- What are you really angry about?

- Can you see any correlation between your anger and your current physical state?

Use your imagination to envisage the physical effects upon the body of years of pent up frustration.

14
Practising Emotions

EMOTIONAL PHYSIOLOGY

If you've identified that you're suppressing, or partially expressing but failing to let go of, one or more emotions, congratulate yourself for being willing to take the risk of keeping an open mind. The following exercises help emotional physiology play a role in your healing. We'll look at anger first.

Anger

Methods of accessing anger are:

1. Hitting a mattress with a soft baton or tennis racquet.
2. Throwing a two year-old temper tantrum.

Precaution 1. If you've never or rarely expressed anger before, the likelihood is that you have some powerful prohibitions to the emotion. One of these is likely to be a consequence of someone "losing it" and hurting someone, an act of violence and not anger as explained previously. This means that your old messages that have kept you safe will be demanding that if you express anger, you are required to hurt yourself or someone else. Your personality or second nature will want you to retreat back into the old adaptations saying.... *"There. I told you so. Anger is dangerous. All that happens is that you get hurt!"* Being aware that this may happen forewarns you. Make sure that you set up the area in which you're going to experiment with allowing anger to happen as safely as possible. Make sure that when you swing a racket or baton you're not going to hurt either yourself or any property of yours that you consider valuable or which in breaking, could hurt you. Check the swing arc of the racquet for objects within it. Wear gloves if your hands are soft. If you're unsure then don't proceed until you are. Do not proceed in the event of you believing that you have a physical condition that would be exacerbated by this, such as a bad back, itself perhaps a consequence of old anger, and a direct consequence of not "backing yourself".

Precaution 2. The two-year-old temper tantrum requires even more care to set up as you'll be lying on your back kicking your legs and hitting your fists into a soft mattress. Make sure that there are no pieces of furniture or other objects which you could kick or punch that would result in you being hurt. The mattress needs to be firm enough to absorb the blows without your heels banging too hard into the floor, but soft enough so that you don't get hurt. A piece of stiff foam rubber, at least six inches thick, is generally good. In addition you need to take into account your physical condition. If you're suffering from a back complaint or any physical ailment that might in your view be exacerbated by doing the two-year old temper tantrum, or the racquet workout, then don't proceed. You may decide that you need another person at the foot of the mattress armed with other soft cushions to keep you from coming off the mattress if the temper tantrum takes over.

Method 1. Kneel on the mattress or just off one end of it. Take a soft baton or a tennis racquet and lift it above your head with two hands, bringing it down upon the mattress. Start very slowly and lightly, getting used to the movement and the sound. A tennis racquet makes a satisfying whack. At the same time open your mouth wide and let out a noise. Start off slowly, gradually increasing the strength of both the hit and the noise. Explore the strength and the frequency of the hits and yells until you become aware of an energy within you that's trying to free itself. To begin with, you may be experiencing some apprehension that may gradually give way to an expression of anger. You don't have to achieve anything with this exercise. Explore allowing the anger to come up. You can come back to it later. On the other hand you may notice to your surprise that the anger flows very freely and takes on a life of its own. It may seem as though, apart from providing the vehicle of its release, it has little to do with you personally, nor, for that matter, what you believed you were angry about.

Method 2. Having cleared a safe space for yourself, lie on your back and gradually start hitting the mattress with your fists, one after the other, left...right....left.....right. Make sure that you can't possibly hit any object within the arc of your fists or legs. You can keep your eyes open or closed. Increase the speed of hitting your fists into the mattress and as you begin to achieve a rhythm with this movement, begin to kick into the mattress with your legs. Keep your legs relatively stiff, with little knee bending whilst you get started. Begin slowly at first and then gradually speed up. You now have to co-ordinate the movements of your fists and your legs. There's a natural movement that at first feels very strange, but as the movement itself takes over from the mechanical way in which you've established it, you may feel the most natural feeling. As the movement becomes more co-ordinated you may notice that your head begins to move rhythmically with the rest of your body. You may notice a side to side movement of your whole body, and you will feel the urge to call out, to yell. Allow this to happen, and let the volume increase naturally. Don't try and yell. Allow the yell to surface from deep down in your psyche wherein it has remained trapped for all these years. You don't need to teach yourself how to do it. Provide the circumstances in which it can happen and you'll be surprised at how natural and easy it feels when the anger....in its own good time....... arises.

DEBRIEFING

One of the reasons we suppressed anger in the first place was because of its association with physical harm. It was implied to us, or directly taught, that anger resulted in someone getting hurt. Anger that is not natural and which has revenge or retribution as its aim, is a calculated anger.....anger intended to harm. This is not anger, the naturally occurring healthy emotion, but another human behaviour that looks similar to anger, called violence. Note the difference between a hoodlum beating someone up and the natural expression of anger in an animal warning another not to invade its territory. In the case of the hoodlum, there's a calculation to the violence that is obvious to an observer. The pathology within such a person's mind is clear. A similar set to the face occurs whenever any psychopath sets out to harm another person, whether physically or mentally. In the case of the animal roaring or hissing at an intruder, the spontaneous show of ferocity is not intended to harm.... but to warn. When an animal hurts another animal in hunting, the emotion, if there is one, appears to be more reverence than anger.

Anger is an emotion distrusted by many in society who have failed to make the distinction between anger with no object and anger with an object. This lack of distinction creates a non-discerning antagonism to any display of anger. This book doesn't focus upon the pros and cons of controlling anger in society, but is vitally interested in freeing us from restrictions to emotional expression, so that we might heal ourselves.

Be aware of your thoughts before, during and after the anger release.

The anger release will free a whole range of thoughts you may be familiar with and more you will have forgotten from the past. Try not to edit any of them. All thoughts are welcome, however critical of you or others they may be. Recall that:

There's no point editing or trying to change your thoughts.

They cannot be changed by you.

They are not yours to change.

You're being "thunk". The Universe is thinking through an agency of itself....you. The thoughts are a natural consequence of the collision of the path you've been travelling and the current circumstances. The current stimuli are registered by your five senses and trigger an old response. If you put any sentient human being through your particular set of conditions and placed him in the circumstances in which you now find yourself, he would be having exactly the same thoughts as you are. They are not aberrant. They are normal for those circumstances. Of course, because those past and present circumstances have never been duplicated before and never will again, the thoughts are unique to the thinker.

Thoughts aren't true and they aren't untrue.

There's no platform from which they can be judged.

They cannot be extrapolated to apply to another set of circumstances. Let them come and visit, and like the good host you are, welcome them, and make them feel at home. After a while they'll have satisfied the reason for their visit and like all natural and good guests they'll take their leave and depart. You will be better for their visit. You can say nothing sensible about them and they warrant no judgement. Thank them for coming. Soon the next visitor will be knocking on your door.

The Objects of Anger

There is no object of anger that is fully released. Anger is a biological response to a stimulus, just like thirst. You're not thirsty with someone or something. It's is a biological request demanding satisfaction. Anger is the same. Its biological intention is part of fight or flight, and it arises as a consequence of fear.

You can use an object to focus upon if the anger seems unwilling to arise. The object may be a physical object, a situation, a person or an entity. You'll know that the physiological first nature anger has taken over from the second nature defensive anger when the object you selected disappears during the release. If the object of your anger remains during the yelling and hitting phase of either workout, you need to return to the mat at a later point. Don't try and force it. The anger has been with you in its modified form for a long while and it's unreasonable to expect it to change overnight.

It may take some years for us to achieve a healthy relationship with our own anger. Until then we maintain objects of anger, someone or something to be angry with, abusing them or us, blaming them or us, making them or us wrong as a way of denying our own guilt, and below the guilt, our own fear and anger. Illness, and often the people we attend to assist us, doctors and others, provide convenient scapegoats for our anger.

And what are we really...really...angry about?

That no-one loved us perfectly in the first place.....and no-one loves us perfectly now.

And what's the fear underlying that anger?

If we're not loved perfectly.....how do we survive?

The principal fear is for our own survival, the most powerful of all fears.

Approximately 15 years of childrearing, unique amongst animals, recasts this fear into our personality. Our responses to life thereafter are dictated by what we've become in order to best accommodate this early childhood fear. Our responses have become "second nature".

"Human nature" is what our collective personalities are commonly termed.

Underneath "human nature" and "second nature" lies "first nature".

15
FEAR

Man is afraid because he's mortal and he faces the unknown.

He's orbiting somewhere, where exactly he hasn't a clue, in a totally unknown direction, for reasons beyond his understanding, and not of his own choosing. Since he created none of his own Universe, he makes up all sorts of fanciful stories to accommodate his ignorance, desperate to avoid the impotence and the fear of simply not knowing. No wonder he's afraid and no wonder he's a master of his own deception, hiding behind fictions and self-delusions that he declares to be truths, often "scientific" truths, whilst pretending to be in control.

Fear is a healthy emotion and needs to be exercised like all other biological systems.

The denial of fear and the masking of fear cause chronic fear or anxiety to develop, leading to disease.

Controlling our fears has been one of the principal preoccupations of mankind, and much of this effort has been directed towards removing fear using drugs, meditations, religious practice, self-hypnosis, self-delusion and many other techniques. However, the way to the peace of mind we seek may not be through the destruction of fear, or the denial of fear, but through the expression of fear. In the expression of fear and the release of fear, peace is temporarily created. The fear will soon re-appear, because, like hunger and thirst, fear is a natural biological phenomenon. Here are a few techniques for reacquainting ourselves with this, one of our most persistent emotional companions.

The first thing is to allow fear to arise incrementally. Take it in small doses – there's no point in being scared out of your wits to the point of being unwilling to explore further. This exploration of fear...... and all other matters we're canvassing in our m3health Program..... never ends, so hurrying doesn't help.

Technique 1. Sit in front of a mirror and imagine you're an actor in a horror movie and you've been asked to portray fear. Experiment with the facial expressions, the noise, the grimaces and your breathing. Start slowly at first and gradually build up the energy and let go a scream. Don't force it. It will arise in its own good time. Repeat this time and again.

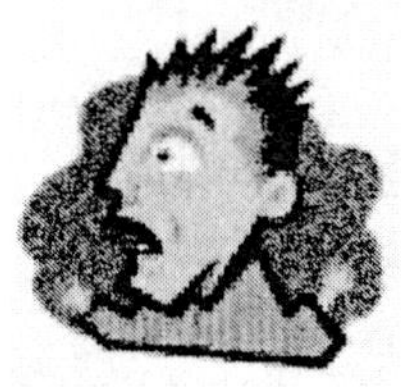

Technique 2. Take a roller coaster ride. If you're a person who's been unwilling to experience fear it's unlikely you'll have frequented amusement parks. There's some really frightening rides these days. Someone who's unwilling to allow fear to arise and to let it go will feel nauseous and may vomit on a scary ride. You must scream. That's why the folks you see riding these things are yelling their heads off. It turns the fear into excitement. Start with the less scary rides first. If you have a medical condition that you believe will be worsened by the physical demands of the ride – use caution and common sense.

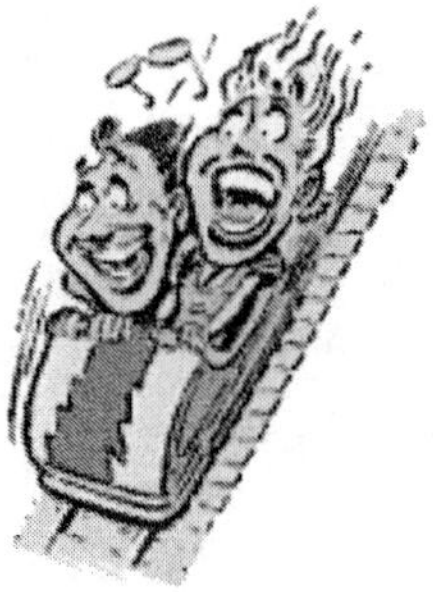

Technique 3. Take in a scary movie or video. If you're seriously fearful of such movies then watch it with a friend.

Technique 4. Use a phobia to get in touch with your fear. A phobia is heightened fear that has become attached to a particular object, such as snakes, spiders or heights. Imagine that you're in the presence of whatever frightens you. If you can set it up safely, and only then, you may consider using your actual phobia to get in touch with your fear.

The expression of fear involves shaking and trembling, as well as the wide eyes, fast pulse and sweating of the typical fight or flight response. You may vomit or need the sudden use of your bowels. Set up your circumstances carefully so that you have the environment in which you can explore your fears. Remember, this is another exercise that will take time to fully realise itself.

The idea is not to get rid of fear...you may as well try and get rid of thirst.... but to enter into a new relationship with fear.

Ultimately, the expression of fear as a means to health and the philosophy of learning to live with fear merge, and I leave it up to others more learned in this matter than myself to offer assistance. Try reading J. Krishnamurti's wonderful little book *Freedom from the Known* for one of the most eloquent treatises on fear. But has anything more vibrant or poignant than Bhagwan Shree Rajneesh's(2) comments on fear ever been written?

"When moments of fear come what to do?

Why should you ask to do anything?

When moments of fear come

be fearful,

tremble with fear,

allow fear to

take possession.

---

2. Bhagwan Shree Rajneesh. *Dying for Enlightenment*. Gunther, Harper & Row, 1979.

Why this constant inquiry,
What to do?
Can't you allow life
in any way to
take possession of you?

When fear comes,
tremble like a leaf
in a strong wind,
and it will be beautiful.
When it has gone
you will feel so serene
and calm,
as when a strong
storm passes by,
everything is left calm
and quiet after it.
Why be always
fighting something?
Fear comes.
It is natural,
absolutely natural.

Allow fear,
don't fight with it.
Watch what is happening,
Go on watching

As your watching eye
becomes more penetrating and intense,
the body will be trembling,
the mind will be trembling.
Deep within you
will be a consciousness
which is simply a witness,
which only watches"

Ah....and you thought that the m3health Program had no poetry....

16
SADNESS

Many of us can hide our anger and fear, but it seems harder to try and hide sorrow. Perhaps we're not so concerned about appearing sad. Either way, most of us can tell when someone is being sad even though the person may be trying to "put on a brave face". If the sadness is long-term the changes to the face become anatomical, and the individual appears permanently sad, even during periods of joy.

Recall that at the same time the observable face is becoming permanently affected by an emotion, in this case sadness, so too the internal organs are physiologically and anatomically impacted. This is the thesis of the book *Love Your Disease : It's Keeping You Healthy* by John Harrison, and is also the basis of the m3health program.

Acute sadness is easier for women and children to express and generally more problematic for men who have powerful social sanctions that reflect poorly upon their manhood should they cry. In an evolutionary sense, it may have been unsafe for men to cry in the midst of life threatening situations in which anger was more suitable to the survival of themselves and the tribe. Whatever the reasons, men often have difficulty shedding tears and this may result in long-term upper respiratory problems including sinusitis, rhinitis, conjunctivitis and blepharitis (inflammation of the margins of the eyelids).

New claims about the value of crying to health suggests that tears have anti-bacterial properties.

There's nothing quite as satisfying as a good cry, best taken as far as men are concerned out of sight of those with whom they'll be doing business tomorrow.

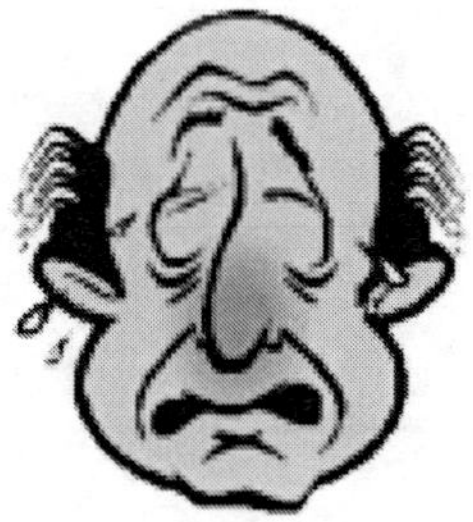

Women tend to like crying together as a method of sharing common feelings and establishing intimate connections.

TECHNIQUE

If you have difficulty crying, create private circumstances where you can experience sadness, the classic and most easily accessible being a good "tear jerker" movie or video. If you go to the cinema sit up the back with a small pack of tissues. Don't force it, for it will come. Ask around and people will let you know what movies make them cry. Those involving children are often good for starters, for they invoke the left over sadness of the little boy or little girl within us.

What are you crying about?

It seems that any current circumstance will enable us to access our long-standing sorrows. We see a small child devastated by the loss of his parents and we cry deep wells of sadness from the very core of our being, from a time long ago when the small child who was us was defenceless, frightened and crying. That core of sadness lives within us, looking always for a conduit to the surface, always searching for someone to heal that old pain.

Only the reader can nurture the child within.

17
JOY

Much is currently being made of the role of joy in the health of the individual.

An "evidence based" scientific paper declares joy is vital to health and by inference, we are now at liberty to believe it. Now that it's been "scientifically validated", and "evidence based", it's changed from untrue to true! What! That doesn't make it valid. It simply adds one minor branch of human exploration, the scientific branch, to a huge old tree of human understanding, an organic understanding if you like. But I digress.

It's so easy to get caught up in the daily routine of work, family pressures, finances, children etc. and turn everything into drudgery. There's joy to be had in all the above and in practically everything else. Putting the joy into things is called "en-joying" them.

The first step of any turnaround is the recognition that something needs to be different. This usually means that something is not being accepted. More of this later. A little stocktaking in respect of the enjoyment in our lives is usually sufficient to change things, but we may need to pencil in those tennis games or that night at the movies, or the babysitter once a fortnight or whatever will free us up a little. If we're locked up by our current problems, illness being one of them, we might do this simple exercise.

TECHNIQUE

Jump up in the air and shout Wheeeeeeeeeee.................

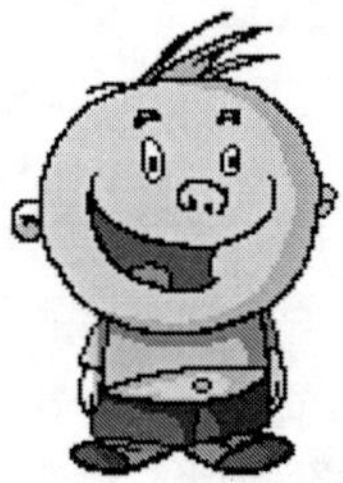

What.....That's it????

Yep....

Keep practising it until a feeling of joy begins to surge through you and takes you over. Joy needs to be given its head and given its heart. Those of you with children can observe it first hand. Children are frequently overtaken with joy, the most wonderful thing to behold. In the case of adults, the shedding of some of our inhibitions is needed to allow the joy to reach us, to flow in a way that contributes to the healing energy.

Over time unbridled joy shapes the immune response, making a contribution to healing. No one thing is responsible for healing, and no one person's healing can be replicated in another. That's why the m3health Program is a companion healer, needing to be adapted and used in ways that the reader believes will help him personally. That said, joy is an integral part of healing.

18
Feral Healer

Imagine that the trappings of the 3rd millennium are fading in your mind and in their place a connection with an ancient place is arising. This connection is just beginning and you're its witness, moving between your new sophisticated brain and your old brain, millions of years in the making.

You're called back down a lost tunnel through the layers of socialisation, through years of "looking good" to the raw essence of who you are. You stand before your first nature whilst your second nature calls you annoyed and anxious..... back to the "real world". The streets call you from their pavements of gold.... the real estate and the cars, the holidays and the halls of fame beckon you back, laughing at your folly. A flicker of recognition that you're not these trappings keeps you searching, but whatever might take their place has not yet formulated for it's no more than a fledgling voice, perhaps even a false prophet. There's enough of you left however to hear the call and you're attracted to it in a way you can't explain. As though the jungle, the desert, the source of the river are all calling your name. You come, tentatively at first but you come nonetheless, frightened, angry even at receiving the call, angry at the messenger and unforgiving of the circumstances. Often through gritted teeth, mostly unwillingly, you come, for what else is there to do. You've tasted the glory, such as it is, and you've found it wanting. You've scaled the heights and found them lower than you imagined and at the top a lot of pressure to stay there or give up and ultimately be judged a failure. You yearn for the time before judgement, before the failure, before the pretence became second nature and consumed you. And now, at this late stage as you face your own mortality you must reconsider, albeit begrudgingly, the beginning. You face the return with trepidation but your instincts are there to guide you and you must let them, perhaps for the first time, have their head. They may lead you to the river of gold, they may lead you to the heart of darkness, they may push you where you swore never to go, whatever happened.

And yet here you are, knocking upon the door of your own self, asking to be let in, for within the defences, underneath the ego lie the old ways, the old mechanism which drives the engine of your soul. Those elements of yourself long denied need now be consulted, for the long adaptation to acceptability has not removed the source, and now it is the source that you need. Approach with respect for within these walls lies the ancient heart, pumping the life force of the universe through your veins as it has always done, despite your best efforts to deny it. The life force gives you the energy, provides you with the inner fire, releases the senses to fulfil your destiny. Here you will find the salvation for which you ache. Here is the way you lost so long ago. Healing awaits you here, for the ancient heart is in touch with Gaia, is in touch with Gondwanaland, is in touch with the Long White Cloud, the warm soft Asian wind, the flutes of the Andes and the African drums. It cannot help but come when called, for it's none other than you.

Within the bosom of your own creation lies a healing force so potent, so alive, so ready and so capable that whatever you do, it simply stands and waits. For no path you have travelled and no illusions you have created can ever take it from you. You have arrived at its door. Soon you will step over the threshold and ask it to heal you, the purpose for which it has always existed. You will re-acquaint yourself with the essence and within the re-union will arise your healing.

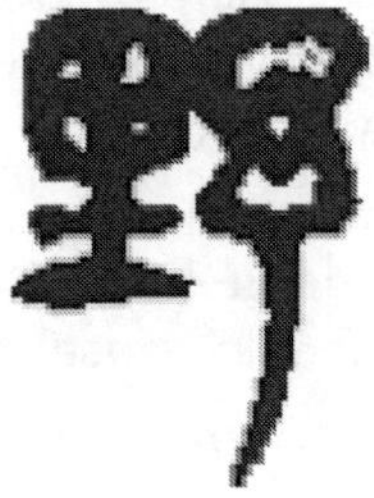

19

HALFWAY REVIEW

Remember how when you decided to take up golf or karate, you were introduced first to the moves.... and some of what you were told made sense, but you were not sufficiently practised to be effective. At that time there was nothing to be done but keep going...just keep going.....

Remember how years later you came back to some of the fundamentals when you needed a shift in your game, and how you realised that the way you played now, though built upon the early foundation, had acquired a nature of its own. You had become the golfer or the fighter. In your best moments there was no separateness between you and the game.... the dancer had become the dance.

The fundamentals of the m3health Program are thinking and feeling.

Our relationship with our thoughts must evolve if we're to free ourselves and our immune system from their restraints. We must move beyond the prison that they've created for us, the prison of our belief that our thoughts are real and that we create them.... that they are us. Instead we need to allow whatever thoughts we might have to arise unhindered and to pass unhindered, regarding ourselves as the vessel of nature that has been chosen to give those particular thoughts expression. They're neither good nor bad, relevant or irrelevant, helpful or unhelpful, healing or damaging.

Waking birds express the morning by singing. But they are not the morning. The morning is the light of the sun arriving at a point on the Earth's surface because the Earth revolves.

Take a close knit circle of friends who go on a camping trip.

These people constitute the essence of a group. Let's imagine that on arriving at the camping ground they all assign themselves tasks, one collects firewood, another water, whilst another erects the tent and yet others start cooking.

When the group reconvenes around the evening campfire, the members of the group do not acquire identities determined by what tasks they've performed on this particular camping trip. They are integral members of the group, and the particular tasks that have been assigned to them or to which they have assigned themselves are temporary functions that don't influence their membership of the group, or who they are.

Thoughts are temporary occurrences made inevitable by the meeting of an organism's past conditioning and current circumstances. Whoooosh...what was that.....oh yes, "I wonder if I'll ever recover"..... I'm remembering my uncle's statement when I was five years old that "Generally people don't recover". This thought has collided with my current illness. Thank you. Next thought please......

Similarly feelings are meant to be experienced, expressed and discharged. That way the organism gets an emotional exercise, not unlike physical exercise, both forms of exercise necessary to keep vital energies flowing. The alternatives are emotional starvation and emotional obesity, neither of which are conducive to good health.

20
Moving Right Along

This page serves the purpose of reminding you to allow yourself the time required for new realisations to settle. Over many years people have reported that each time they review the m3health material they take another step. Our psyches are only capable of so much assimilation at any one time, and body physiology has to unlearn and then re-learn.

There's no time frame better than any other.

Those of you with a life threatening illness will need to experience the fear which comes from taking your time..... time which you may believe that you don't have. This would be more beneficial than hurrying through the exercises and the pages, believing that once you've reached the end, a magic formula for healing will be revealed.

The best opportunity for healing is to get the mind and body thinking, feeling, experiencing and doing in ways that are conducive to healing rather than disease. Then the time frame is up to nature.

It's impossible to predict the "correct" course of action, or the correct sequence of realisations, because no-one knows.

No two people are alike and no person is the same today as he was yesterday.

Experiment with allowing something.......you may not know what.....to dictate your next move.

Explore being available for something unexpected to arise. If elation arises, bring it into the program. If frustration or a belief that you're not progressing arises, it too must be allowed its time in the light.

21
Doing

A good friend of mine, an inveterate seeker and visitor to India came across a flyer indicating that the celebrated sage Jiddha Krishnamurti was to give a speech at a local hall. The flyer said:

"DO NOT ASK ME WHAT TO DO"

Tonight 7p.m. - 9p.m.

Town Hall

a talk by J. Krishnamurti

Not long into the evening the audience became very agitated when several people, ignoring the title and the obvious thrust of the speech, asked their master what they should do to live more fulfilling lives. When Krishnamurti replied that he did not know what they should do, the hall erupted and the Police were forced to move in and close the meeting down to prevent a riot.

As the speaker was being jostled by the crowd and ushered out of the hall several people were seen by my friend to be clinging onto the robes of the master and imploring him...... "Master, master.....Won't you please tell us what to do."

Then there's the story of the man with 12 children who approached Bhagwan Shree Rajneesh saying, "Master, I have 12 children and cannot feed them, what can I do?"

"Do!"........replied Rajneesh, "Do"!......... "Haven't you *done* enough already!"

Human Beings have a particular fondness for the belief that *doing* something is the essence of change, a belief engendered by the fear of the opposite—doing nothing and trusting in nature, or as Rajneesh said, "allowing life to take possession of you". Nature has been superseded as the doer of mighty deeds, and now medicine and technology reign supreme at the top of the league of achievers of great outcomes or miracles.

However, as well as addressing what needs to be done, it might be equally important to address the doer, rather than only the thing he's doing. The notion of doing something vs. doing nothing is a valuable exploration, for we in the Western countries have been raised on a diet of doing as opposed to being. We prize doing highly, whilst we almost universally discount being. The prizes of Western society and most societies for that matter are based on the "doer wins" principle, epitomised in the exhortation to anyone in trouble......... "Well, what are you going to do about it!" "He's a doer", we cry, in adoration and exultation of the deeds of the successful, measured by how much money they have, how much status, or even more philanthropically, how many good deeds they've done.

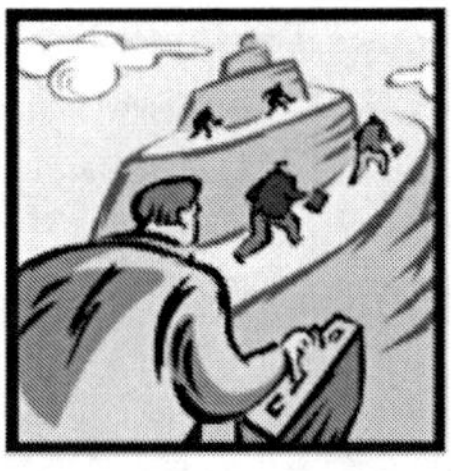

Doing is a vital part of human experience and survival, but not all of it. We have now reached the point in our material evolution where doing may be interfering with allowing and being, and at the same time may equally be interfering with healing. In the desperation to do, healing is once again compromised, for the act of doing may suppress the relationship with our self that is so vital to healing. Many of you will already have experienced the frustration of attending doctor after doctor, therapy after therapy, investigation upon investigation, always trying to do something or have something done to us that will heal us. All the while the inner healer is in abeyance, unwittingly put on hold.

But our healer hasn't gone away, it cannot go away, for nothing we "do" can ever fully suppress it. Like a witness, our inner healer is also a server who only stands and waits. It need not be "doing" anything to be quietly working its magic.

Doing makes up the third of the triumvirate of elements with which the sufferer must contend. The other two are thinking and feeling, much of which has been made elsewhere.

Doing something suppresses the fear of doing nothing. If we leave our healing up to nature, our inner healer, how do we know that it will be effective? We don't. We have no idea if we're capable of the sort of m3health Inquiry that will result in a favourable outcome. It feels a lot safer to either put our self in someone else's hands or do lots of things to help our self. This latter also earns the approval of loved ones who are also suffering at our dilemma and who are also very disconcerted by the prospect of the first nature of the sufferer being unmasked, opening up the family mask to scrutiny. They have become accustomed to relating to the second nature of the person, it's become second nature to them, and they don't want that boat rocked, hence their support for the sufferer doing...doing.... doing.

How do you know what you should be doing?

Here are a few questions to assist.

- Do you feel that you've left no stone unturned in your exploration of this illness?
- What do you think about that?
- What do you feel when you think about it?
- What else could you have done?
- Are you tired of doing things about your disease?
- How would you like things to be different?
- What does the notion of doing nothing bring up for you?
- What feelings does it invoke?

Let everything you think and feel about doing nothing, compared with doing something about your illness arise and be noted.

- Do you know what you should be doing next?
- Does anyone else know what you should be doing next?
- Who's in a position to judge what's best for you?
- Do you have any derogatory or condemnatory voices in your head reporting on your efforts to heal yourself thus far?
- Do you have any negative or positive comments in respect of yourself or healers whom you've engaged in your quest for healing?

Write them down.

Remember our work on thinking. What you say about yourself and about anyone else is an inevitable collision between your past and current circumstances and does not make your beliefs or thoughts true, any more than an oak tree, a quirk of nature, can claim to be truer or more natural than an elm.

What's your response to the following claim?

"What you should be doing is what you are doing."

"What you ought to have done is what you did."

Experiencing the discomfort of doing nothing is an integral part of this process. It might be helpful to review the section on fear.

22
ET TU BRUTÉ

There's a good argument that we criticize ourselves more than we criticize anyone else..... and more than anyone else criticizes us.

These comments even apply to those people who appear to be very critical of others and not of themselves. Unless we're critical of ourselves over something, we're impervious to the criticism of others over the same matter. Similarly we don't criticise others unless we're fearful of being labelled with the same imperfection, and deep down critical of ourselves.

Summarised, a critical person is critical of himself as well as others and a non-critical person criticises neither himself nor others.

Let's re-visit the voice in our head that comments upon us.

That voice may be "negative", or self-congratulatory.

- What do you say about yourself?
- What are your common criticisms of others?

EXERCISE

(a) Become as specific as you can about any criticisms that you make about others........or any critique, "positive" or "negative" which you commonly make about others.

Spend some time doing this, at least five minutes.

Now say them about yourself instead.

Do they fit?

(b) Take each criticism and say it to yourself in the same voice and with the same mannerisms as your mother or father might have criticised you.

Are you able to identify where these criticisms are coming from? Humour me on this one.....Assume that these critiques aren't your own dispassionate, objective judgements, but a simple rote regurgitation of something someone either directly told you or implied indirectly by their own actions, i.e. modelled. And this at a time when you had no way of providing any alternative viewpoint or perspective.

- Are there any people in your life at the moment whose criticisms of you are important to you?
- Who are they?
- Can you identify anyone from your past who your current critics represent?

If your contemporary critic is a representative of someone in your own mind or someone you can identify as a critic from the past (usually mum, dad or both) his or her opinion of you may have increased in significance after the death of one of your parents. Put simply, the person is taking mum or dad's place in your pantheon of critics. For example, men often report that after the death of their own father another man who need not necessarily be older, is cast in the role of critic. The critic may be reluctant, but is held in the man's mind as someone who demands pleasing or measuring up to.

Here's an exercise to determine who might be a critic in your life.

EXERCISE

Imagine that you're about to be awarded the highest honour in your profession or field of endeavour. You're offered two tickets to the presentation ceremony. Who do you invite?

Who came up for you?

These people will often feature in your dreams or when you muse on "making it" in your life in some way, whether it be in business, sport, community service, church service, philanthropy or any other endeavour at which you would like to succeed. Whenever you receive an accolade, they're there in your mind.

Who in your life right now are you keen to impress?

Your past critic can often be identified by examining who you try and impress as a grown up – men or women – young or old?

Self-deception must be addressed and engaged for healing, for only an open minded willingness to inquire, however unpalatable, however frightening and however long it takes, will assist healing. Self delusion and certainty does not facilitate healing.

Nor does enrolling others in those same delusions on the promise of the mutual safety to be found in a fortress like defence of attitudes, opinions, beliefs and matters of which we say, "We're certain".

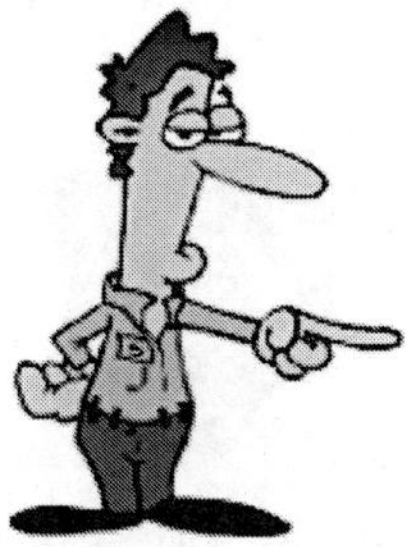

We're identifying influences that have played a part in our condemnation or congratulations of ourselves and others. Some people call this the critical parent in our head. If we're to recover from illness we might need to decommission this critical parent. It matters not whether the criticism is "negative" or "positive". It remains a judgement interfering with our capacity for free thought and an equally free immunological response.

The thoughts need to be dis-engaged from the biological organism, the temporary host whom they're visiting, whatever the thoughts may be and whomever their host.

We benefit from accepting the thoughts, not changing them.

This is the opposite of resigning oneself to the validity and the truth or universality of the thoughts. When we welcome our thoughts as visitors with little impact upon our first nature, they leave us. This is tantamount to self-acceptance.

Accepting our self:

Whoever we are

However we are

Wherever we are

Whenever we are

Such self-acceptance is not something which we do, but something which we explore. During our exploration, self-acceptance gradually shows up, but when it does, we won't recognise it, for it's moved on from being of consequence. We generally need an outsider to point out to us any change in our acceptance of ourselves.

"Boy, you're way less tough on yourself these days. Do you realise that?"

"Well, no".... we reply,...... "but now you come to mention it........."

23
Cause and Cure

There are many factors that "cause" illness. With every new scientific advance a new cause is postulated. Then repetition turns theory into fact and all other causes are consigned to the dustbin reserved for quacks and charlatans. This, much of the time, is "science" at work.

It's more likely that "causes" are contributing agents, rather than explanations of a single disease origin. The causal agents are inter-related in such a way as to make isolation of them non-contributory. For example, a genetic pre-disposition to a disease may not result in an expression of the disease unless another set of preconditions are met, the epigenome.

Some causal agents are obvious.

For example, smoking a packet of cigarettes a day isn't helping chronic bronchitis and needs to be stopped before the body can begin to repair the damage in susceptible individuals. On the other hand plenty of people smoke a packet of cigarettes a day and never get bronchitis, or anything else for that matter. So smoking in one person is a definite causal agent in bronchitis and definitely not in another. This is different from the blanket statement "Smoking causes bronchitis".

There are plenty of statistics to demonstrate that "Smoking causes cancer" as all cigarette packets inform us.

However, this may be oversimplifying the case. That smoking cigarettes and lung cancer are related is beyond statistical dispute. But does that mean that one "causes" the other? Perhaps it means that people who are attracted to smoking cigarettes are also likely to suffer from lung cancer for reasons yet to be determined? Perhaps they're more nervous than other people and their neurotransmitters lead them to smoke for relief of anxiety. At the same time their high levels of adrenalin and cortisone create abnormal lung cells. Perhaps a particular gene is damaged by smoking in some people and impervious to smoking in others.

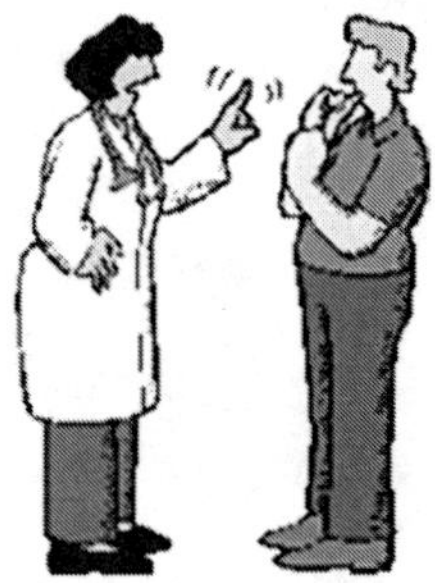

Causes of diseases are not as straightforward as some proponents would have us believe. That's why I prefer to use the term "causal agent". No two people respond identically to a causal agent.

Common sense must prevail, as well as taking into account the general case. Common sense tells us that inhaling a large amount of smoke is not going to be good for our lungs, whatever the statistics tell us.

Intuition tells us that we're unlikely to get rid of the 'flu this winter if we keep smoking cigarettes.

Much of the time the causal agents are far harder to identify than in the case of cigarettes and lung conditions.

Genetics, womb environment, early childhood conditioning, schooling, community social values, diet, pollution, stress, physical environment and evolution all play their role in the cause and cure of disease. Everyone is different. No two personalities or sets of defences are the same. No two biologies are the same and it's highly unlikely that any two causal agents in any two people will result in the same disease manifestation.

What does this mean for those of us trying to heal ourselves?

It means that your m3health Inquiry will be different from that of all others.

Whatever your particular combination of nature and nurture, it's unique.

Health and recovery occur when your unique physiology is re-united with your unique healing circumstances.

Because we've lost contact with what these may be, we need to become explorers again.

We can use whoever is available to help, but part of this exploration is ours to make alone.

In undertaking the m3health Program, it helps to use yourself as the example.

24
SELF ACCEPTANCE

Acceptance of ourselves is not highly regarded in many societies where it's believed that self-criticism is preferable.

Ongoing self-analysis and criticism is regarded as good for developing powerful, self-reflective personalities. Many of us don't differentiate between acceptance of ourselves and self-aggrandisement, self-congratulation or, in the popular vernacular, "having tickets" on ourselves. However, acceptance implies no criticism, either positive or negative. The person who is self-accepting has nothing to say about himself, and nothing to say about others either.

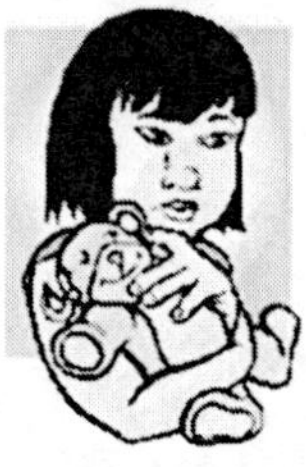

Children are encouraged or bullied by grown ups into conforming to society's rules "for their own good", and the main weapon in this assault is to be critical of the child and encourage him to be critical of himself. "For their own good" means to be acceptable to their tribe or community. The alternative is regarded as indulging a child who grows up hedonistic and incapable of feeling for others. Instilling a good dose of guilt is considered necessary for both the children and the community. Without guilt, what would stop everyone from simply pleasing himself, without regard for the well-being of others?

Tit for tat strategies in "reciprocal altruism" suggest that human beings are best served by treating their fellow man well. Tit for tat basically says that you assume another person will do the right thing by you and the tribe until shown otherwise. This provides a measure of insurance that you'll be treated well in return, and under such mutually agreed principles the tribe flourishes. If one's fellow man does not treat you well then you're free to treat him badly, for you must take the necessary steps to protect yourself, and he's already proven himself to be a danger to you and possibly to the tribe.

In this scenario it's difficult to see how a person would benefit from self-criticism. It would appear un-biological, since the person in a reciprocally altruistic set of circumstances would need to stand up for himself and could not afford the consequences of self-criticism. Under the burden of his own criticism he may become slow to act in his own interests, deferring out of guilt to the interests of others instead.

In this instance both he and the tribe would suffer because both could be held to ransom by an individual who, for any reason of biological variance, failed to live by the rules, thereby jeopardizing the common interest in favour of his own.

Excessive self-criticism might not only be a liability to the safety of both the afflicted individual and his tribe, but a personal liability to his own well-being, mediated via an immune system restricted in its natural efforts to fight off invaders and remedy internal malfunctions. The immune system is best served by regarding invaders who are not proved friendly, as hostile.

And so our excessively self-critical individual is inviting trouble.

How can someone who's full of criticism move from beneath such a yoke?

We must go back to the principle of thoughts and feelings.

The self-critical thoughts are best welcomed, noted, and allowed to pass freely through the organism.

"What was that?" You inquire of another self-attack.

"What?..... I'm a waste of space!"

"I hear you..... thanks for visiting. Come again soon."

Of course, were this to be your actual relationship with a critical thought, it may be the last critical thought you ever had!

There's no point in trying to change thoughts, you can't any more than you can personally change the orbit of the moon. Identifying with them is the problem, not the thoughts themselves. In other words it's the "I" in "I'm no good" which is causing the problem. You're "I"-dentifying with what you regard as your "I", or your ego. And yet this is simply the record of your journey – your life passport if you like. It indicates which part of experience and existence has been assigned to the particular biological organism you call "me".

Don't bother trying to change what you say about yourself. You may as well try and change your parents, or the house you lived in when you were five years old.

Consider how you'd feel if someone wanted to throw out all your old family photos. There may be precious few of them.... some of them from good times....others you'd rather forget..... but you don't want to throw them out and replace them with someone else's instead. What would be the point? We'd reject the offer to replace our family photos with others in which the subjects smile more.

What you say about yourself and others is a bit like the old family photos, an accurate record of where you've been. Painful though some of them are, you still like to drag them out and look at them once in a while. You're no longer that child in those photos...but that's certainly who you used to be.

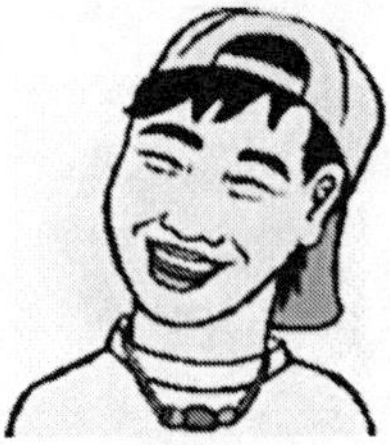

Acknowledgement of the journey and the thoughts and feelings which are a consequence of the journey is enough to move you beyond them. The feelings need to be allowed to fulfil their biological function by completing themselves. The thoughts will do the same thing over time.

Your role is to allow the thoughts and feelings to resolve themselves, whilst you learn to accept yourself doing nothing.

“How hard can that be?”......I hear you ask.....

Hmmm......good question.

25
JUDGEMENT

Judgement is the process whereby we make comment upon our self, others or any other matter. It includes both positive and negative criticism, although the term "criticism" has more recently been given a negative connotation.

Where does judgement come from?

We like to think of ourselves as "good judges of character" or a "good judge of people", capable therefore of knowing what's really going on. The more energy we invest in the judgement, the greater the need of the critic for the safety which judgement affords. Far from being an independent assessment, the judgement is designed primarily to protect the judge. Of course the judgements are accurate and often impressive because the judge acquired them under great duress as a child – that's why he's so good at them. Often the judgements are meant to put others on the back foot, using attack as the best method of defence.

The judgement is triggered by a contemporary event, not of our making. The judgement is a visitation from the past, not of our making. So why would we congratulate ourselves about the accuracy and observation of our judgements? They're mostly a cry for help from someone who needed to acquire them in the first place.

The suspension of judgement is the freeing of the mind, the body, the soul and the immune system

The way to suspend judgement is to allow judgement

Allowing judgement recognises it for what it is, a defence mechanism. Allowing judgement, and not attacking ourselves for needing to acquire it in the first place, decommissions it.

And what happens when judgement is exhausted, when thoughts, feelings and actions come and go unfettered by the need to judge and criticise them?

A state of being replaces judgement.

Doing

Thinking **without judgement = being**

Feeling

26
Being

What's going to replace the traffic in my head if I stop hanging onto old beliefs and partially expressed emotions?

Some of us have never experienced a quiet mind, let alone a silent mind.

Nature lovers come closest when they're in communion with their favourite place, be it the mountains, the beach, the bush, the ocean, a flower or a baby.... That state of completeness or contentment where the witness and the experience are without boundaries...... where the response is uncontaminated by judgement......where the thoughts and feelings flow unhindered.......vibrating the soul....

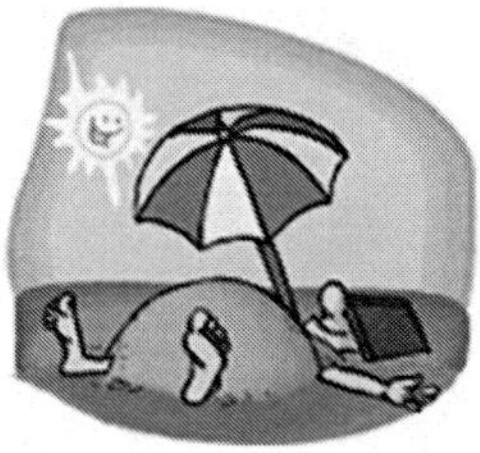

In such circumstances there's nothing to say...for nothing speaks so eloquently of itself.

Most of us have had that experience.

This is the experience of being.

27
SELF

Myself, yourself, himself, herself, itself........what are all these selfs?

Who are they?

Who am I?

Try this exercise:

Describe yourself.

Now take some time over this before you read on.... or are you going through this whole m3health Program as if it has nothing to do with you personally.... as if it doesn't apply to you.....dismissing it as perhaps of value to someone you know, but not applicable to yourself....

Note down what you say about yourself.

What did you put down?

Did you mention your job?

Did you mention your gender, your age, your marital status, how many children you have, your sporting achievements, your address, your nationality, your intelligence, your physical characteristics, your house, your wealth, your investments, your community achievements, your hat size, your car, your title, your........

Difficult to know who you are, isn't it....

Maybe we're none of those things. But what's this got to do with me healing myself.......?

The healing force that waits to rescue you lies within the core, the essence of your being, deep within your "self".

Surrounding it are the acquisitions of living, the defences, the adaptations, the attitudes, beliefs and opinions making up your ego or your personality. They have become second nature, shielding your first nature or your self from the difficulties and the fears of living openly. But they're also keeping you in a state in which you're unable to respond with fifteen million years of healing evolution — they're keeping you from your self.

The adaptations are what we come up with when we try and say who we are.

We're so contrived, so adapted that we no longer know who we are, if we ever did. We stumble along occupied with thoughts that aren't ours, living lives which don't suit us, until something goes horribly wrong and we suddenly wake up to the fact that we're off track. We've lost touch with our self.

We don't know who we are, just who we've struggled to become, struggling for safety whilst imagining it to be a struggle for prosperity and hoping that along with prosperity will come peace and health. But instead what shows up is an increasing separateness and isolation, and an increasing distance from that which heals.

And what does heal? Please try the exercise below.

Cast your mind to a time when you felt at peace or even an exhilaration with the surroundings in which you found yourself.

Be there now in your mind if you will. You may have to sort through various images to come up with one on which you can settle for the time being. You can do this exercise as many times as you like so that it's not important to have the perfect scene.

Allow yourself to be in the scene.

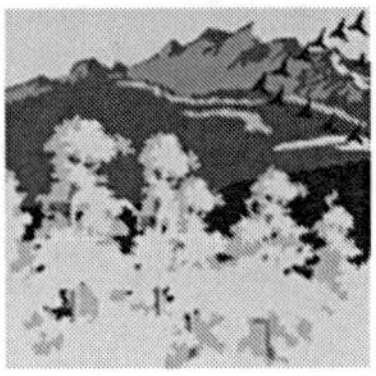

Where are you?

What are you thinking?

What are you feeling?

Is there another person with you or are you alone?

What is it about this place that so affects you?

Describe in detail to yourself your physical location, your surroundings.

The great likelihood is that you're describing an aspect of unaffected nature, a beautiful place or a very natural person, perhaps a child, or an animal unaffected by the defences of personality. You're communing with nature. Your first nature is in communion with nature. You're at one with your surroundings, at one with the Universe.

Do you feel a surge of energy, a zest for life, an exhilaration you may remember from childhood perhaps?

You've allowed your energy and the energy of nature to merge, and to drop the separateness behind which we hide much of the time

You're in the healing zone.

Healing happens when you allow your own life force to access nature. Your immune system gets in touch with nature and together they heal you. This book is an inquiry into the various mechanisms you've used to keep nature and healing away. Now could be the time to get back in touch with nature.

Wow!

How incredibly simple.

One of the most important things for you to do now is to set up circumstances in which you can experience the beauty and the power of nature. Now how do we do that?

We all know of places such as the one you've allowed yourself to return to in your mind. Perhaps the magic can be re-visited. Was it a deserted beach, the rainforest, the desert, the mountains, skiing in perfect powder, riding a wonderful barrel in perfect offshore ten foot conditions, walking the dog through the forest near your house, pottering in the garden, riding the bike around the perimeter of your farm, being outside at night in the middle of nowhere with only the stars for company, making love to your partner, hearing the call of the prairie or the throbbing beat of a primitive dance ceremony, driving across the plains or any other of a million locations and activities or lack of activity that brings you close to nature.

Part of healing is to revisit these places and explore others.

Part of healing is to commune with nature in your mind, as well as with your senses and with your body.

28
MEDITATION

Whoaa.....back off buddy.....I've come along with you so far, somewhat sceptically I might add, but I really don't think that I want to go down the uncertain pathway of eastern philosophy....

Hmmmm...... O.K..... skip this bit.

For the rest of you, let's see if this rather fascinating phenomenon can be of assistance. First of all, what is it? Secondly, how do you do it, if indeed it can be *done*?

Let's start with a suggestion. If you proceed with this and you find that there's something to this meditation caper, you'll be surprised at how familiar it is to you. At the end of our exercise you might well be able to identify when you've previously experienced a similar state.

Was it in childhood? Was it walking down that deserted beach we were speaking of recently? Let's find out.

To begin our exploration of meditation it might be helpful to review the characteristics of an inquiry. Principally, an inquiry, including the m3health Program, doesn't try and achieve anything. Healing is revealed in the course of the m3health Program – the inquiry is the healing medium. After the program you'll be unable to say exactly what happened. More particularly you'll be unable to instruct anyone else in taking the same journey, since yours will not heal him and his journey will not heal you.

There are no lessons to be learned, only lessons to be taken

This can be pretty infuriating since most of us have been taught that we learn by watching others. And many times this works. But it won't work this time, because you must go where nobody, yourself included.....has been before.

Meditation has a lot in common with the m3health Inquiry.

As Rajneesh said:

"A Master is not someone who's achieved anything.

A Master is someone who's learned that there's nothing to achieve."

However, the achievement of nothing may be some achievement indeed.

But I digress.

Meditation, like healing, must be allowed to come, not forced to come.

Meditation techniques are designed to pass the time whilst waiting to heal. The techniques take the conscious mind out of the equation allowing the natural healing mechanisms of the body to do their job. Here's one of them. Please forgive my simple attempts at explaining what many believe takes a pupil a lifetime of practice to achieve. There are as many theories and principles of meditation as there are of medicine and more – probably as many as there are people on the Planet who've ever meditated. If you get interested in this practice and feel the need for more detailed instruction please speak to others or consult a meditation teacher, far more practised in the meditative arts than myself. Meanwhile, here's a few suggestions to begin with.....take it easy.

See the Caution at the end of this section before you attempt the meditation

EXERCISE

Set up a room in which you won't be interrupted. Turn off all appliances that might interfere with a state of relaxation, and lock the door if you don't want anyone to disturb you. Don't tell other people that you're trying this just yet — it doesn't help — but it does hinder.

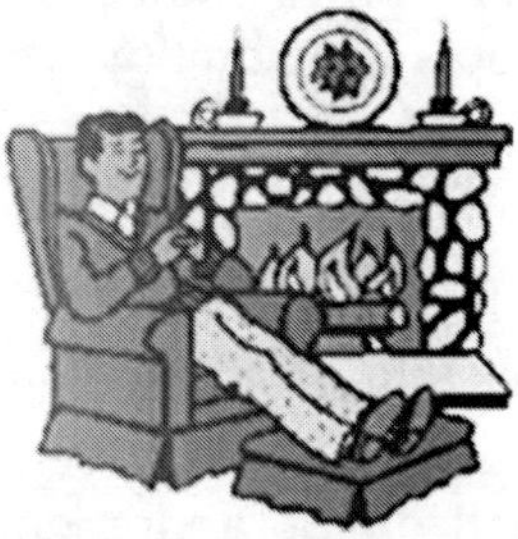

Sit in whatever position you feel inclined to, from cross legged (lotus position) to sitting in a comfortable chair. There are many principles of how to sit. For our purposes I'm ignoring them in favour of the "make yourself comfortable" edict. You can even lie down if you prefer, but it makes it more difficult to stay awake and alert.

Sit for a few moments, doing nothing in particular. During the course of our m3health Inquiry you've acquired significant experience in identifying the fact that you are, in actuality, thinking, and you've become somewhat practised in observing your thoughts — ***noting*** them is the term we've been using. As you sit quietly one thing is highly likely — you will be breathing.

Take notice of your breath. When you breathe, your diaphragm, that large sheet of muscle which separates the chest from the abdomen, moves up and down, drawing air into the lungs when it moves towards the abdomen, and pushing air out of the lungs when it moves upward. As it moves upward the contents of your abdomen have more room and your abdomen falls. When you breathe in your diaphragm pushes the contents of your abdomen outwards. Look down at your abdomen now and see if you can notice just such a movement. Yes? No? If the latter, remove the clothing covering your abdomen and look again. Breathe in and notice the movement of your abdomen. Ah ha.... now I see it....but hullo.... it appears to be moving in the opposite direction to that which I'm suggesting. Quite so. It may move in either direction when you breathe in, depending on whether you're breathing primarily using the movement of your chest wall or the movement of your diaphragm. It matters not a jot. The point is that it's moving up and down, rising and falling, depending on how you're sitting or lying, in keeping with the breath.

So we note the movement of, the rise and the fall of... the abdomen.

Rise.......fall......rise......fall.....rise......fall.....rise....

We can now shut our eyes if we haven't already done so and note the rise and fall of the abdomen as we breathe. Some people find it helpful in the first instance to place their hands, or a single hand, upon the abdomen as this assists in identifying the rise and the fall. Proceed as you like.

Don't make any attempt to change your breathing.

Don't try and relax. Don't try and do anything. Consider your normal breathing. You don't try and breathe. It happens automatically, so you don't have to do anything. Simply observe. Just watch the rise and fall of the abdomen.

You're not trying to change or influence your breathing.

By now you may have noticed that as you focus upon the rise and fall of your abdomen your mind wanders. Let it. Don't chastise it or exhort it to stop chattering to you. It doesn't matter what the thoughts are, and believe me, they'll be a varied bunch.... just simply note the fact that you're thinking.

When you notice that your mind has wandered away from noting your breathing, say to yourself, silently, "Thinking... thinking...." Each time you become aware of the fact that you're thinking, use that realisation to return to noting the rise and fall of the abdomen......

Rise....fall....rise....fall....rise....fall.....rise.....fall.....

Keep doing this.

Now you may have noticed something else. You may have noticed that you hear things in the room next door or outside in the street or in the woods. Good. Don't try and do anything about this. Simply note it. "hearing... hearing..." you say to yourself. Once again, use the awareness that you're hearing something to return to noting your breathing......

...rise...fall...rise...fall...rise....fall.

What next might you notice? Well, if you've already been going more than a few minutes, you may well have begun to feel some bodily sensation. Perhaps an itch, or if you're trying to sit cross legged on the floor, a pain, or a burning. Good. Simply note it...."

"Itch....itch, or pain....pain...." and return to the rise and fall of the abdomen.......rise....fall....rise.....fall....rise.....fall.

It may take seconds or minutes before you realise that your mind has again wandered and this time you're looking in your mind at some scene or picture, often associated with thinking. Once again, simply note it, perhaps "seeing....seeing" would suit you, and use the fact that you've become aware of it to once again return to the rise and fall of the abdomen....

...rise...fall...rise....fall....rise....fall.....rise.....fall....rise.....fall....

Break off this practice whenever it suits you. If you keep going you'll probably begin to experience some interesting phenomena. Emotions can arise pretty powerfully in these early stages. Allow them to arise. Don't try and force them up and don't try and force them away. Once again simply note them:

"anger .....anger" or "sadness....sadness" or "joy...joy"... or my favourite, "fear...fear". Use the arrival of the emotions and your recognition of them to return to the breathing....

.....rise...fall...rise...fall....rise....fall....rise....fall....rise

And that's all there is to it. (Howls of protest from experienced meditators noted.) Conventional wisdom would have you meditate twice a day for about half an hour each sitting, but I suggest you try it for as long as it seems to suit you and whenever it suits you.

CAUTION: There's no doubt in my mind after many years of clinical practice that this is a powerful technique capable of many things, not all of which are agreeable to everyone.

If you're feeling very vulnerable or unsupported at the moment, now might not be the right time to practice meditation. If you're too fearful of the consequences of experiencing something over which you might not have complete control, you may need to review the remainder of this book before you have the confidence to proceed with the meditation.

As with every other suggestion from this book or from anyone else that may affect you, take your time and seek the counsel of anyone whose opinion you value.

Then decide for yourself.

29
FINDING OUR SELFS

This is usually expressed as finding ourselves, typically in a sentence such as ".... wandering along a country path we suddenly found ourselves in the midst of a sea of colourful wildflowers...." or "Finding ourselves late for the show, we made our way back to the hotel..." or "It was a great relief to find oneself surrounded by others in similar circumstances..."

In all of these very different circumstances the language indicates that a person or people got a fix on where they were or what they were doing. Something, anyway...was discovered.

If we take this a bit further and break down the word "ourselves" into "our selfs", i.e. we found our selfs, we have another interesting meaning. In the course of doing something ordinary, our selfs or inner beings reveal themselves....they are found. Is this another instance of original meaning having been superseded by contemporary usage? We've seen several examples of this already.

Disease meaning dis-ease or discomfort is one. Responsibility from response-ability, the ability to respond, is another. Yet another is represent from re-present, to bring back to the present. Finding ourselves or finding our selfs is another, for it indicates that in the course of any activity at all, we can find our self, that elusive core of our being that became hidden behind our personalities.

An essential prerequisite to have our "self" show up in the course of ordinary activity is that we don't go looking for it.

Perhaps we never actually lost it, but for safe keeping surrounded it with the adaptations necessary to survive this existence. Concealed for all that time, it now needs a little freedom if our healing capabilities are to show up.

Freeing of the self is the second phase of our lives, a life in which there are two general periods. The first is the acquisition of the defences. The second is the shedding of the defences. Both are necessary and natural.

The more intellectually we approach healing.... the more we try and do it perfectly.... the more we leave little or nothing to chance, the more we're getting in our own way. Many people interested in a healing Program such as the m3health Inquiry, are successful people accustomed to "making things happen".

They like to control the process.

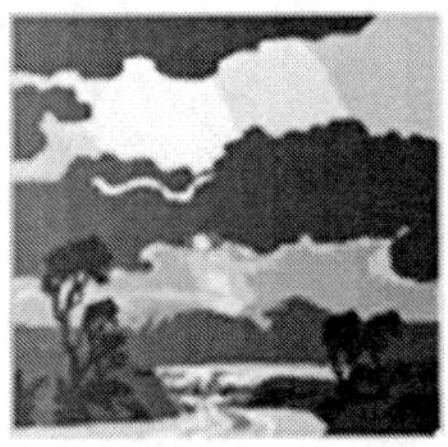

Healing needs to be allowed to happen, not forced to happen.

You can't force healing to happen. You can't control it. The more space you provide for it to show up the more likely it is to happen.

How do I provide space for healing?

Ah.....providing space is not something which you *do*.

Take a moment to be with the discomfort of that realisation.

Recovery demands that you take a back seat to nature, and if you're thinking about back seat driving........forget it!

The delightful thing about "finding our selfs" is that healing could be just around the corner whilst we're pursuing the most mundane activity, and it may well be something we've done or somewhere we've been many times before. A smile in the street from a child, the song of a bird, a soft ocean breeze, a look of love from a partner or the shimmering of the heat in the desert are widely diverse circumstances in which we find ourselves. In such moments we find our selfs, connected with, not separated from, creation.

Your world is full of simple and beautiful healing moments, and you're opening to them like a flower to rain.

If we're seriously ill, our inclination is to follow a course of action that was undertaken by another sufferer who recovered. What could be more understandable? However, in my experience people do better by following their own intuition. If that takes them down an already worn path, fine, but it's more likely that being the unique individual you are, your pathway to health will be similarly unique and untried.

Your journey may seem left field to loved ones and a concern to medical attendants, but you must ultimately travel alone. By all means take the advice of those who you depend upon for safety, but you must also take the risk of allowing your own healing path to declare itself.

It must choose you.

The m3health Program has suggested a strategy for clearing obstacles so that your unique healing strategy can reveal itself.

30
ACCEPTANCE

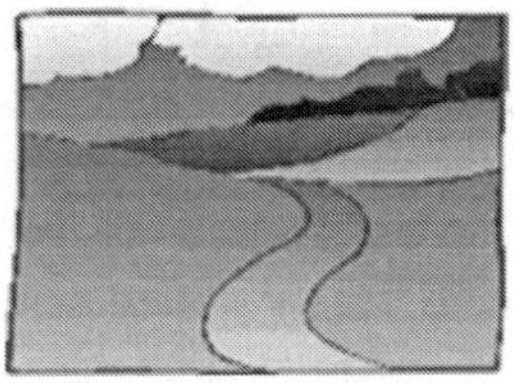

I've often wandered lonely as a cloud

as often as often is

as lonely as lonely can be

as cloudy as cloudy is,

as I as I can be

Concepts of change have occupied many professions in recent times from psychologists to business managers. Mostly in considering change we get caught up in concepts of power, ego, courage, judgement and "shoulds and oughts". Of course, we want to control it.

Reinhold Niebuhr wrote:

"God, give us grace to accept with serenity the things that cannot be changed, courage to change the things that should be changed, and the wisdom to distinguish the one from the other."

At times we may be trying a bit too hard to stay in control of the change process, for we may not always know what should be changed.

Another way of approaching change is to "allow" change to happen rather than trying to "make" it happen. This suggests that things won't change unless they're accepted, and also that the very act of accepting them guarantees that they will change, since nothing stays the same for long.

It may not be possible for human beings to know how things "should" be. It's impossible obtaining consensus, and added to the fact that we're hurtling around in space in the middle of we wouldn't know where as a consequence of we wouldn't know what for reasons utterly beyond our comprehension, it's a little ridiculous trying to control an outcome, when you think about it. We haven't even got a clue what the best outcome might be, let alone have the power to achieve it!

Acceptance is dynamic. It does not mean inactivity. Neither does it mean resignation.

Acceptance means thinking, feeling and doing something, without the need to ruminate about it, without the need to judge it. It means allowing outcomes, not dictating them.

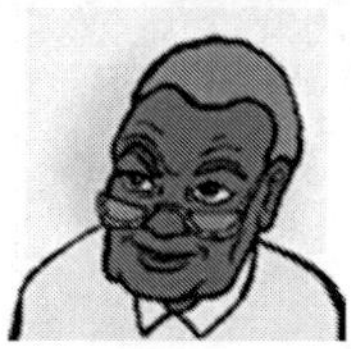

Accept Everything....

Change Nothing.....

and

Everything Changes

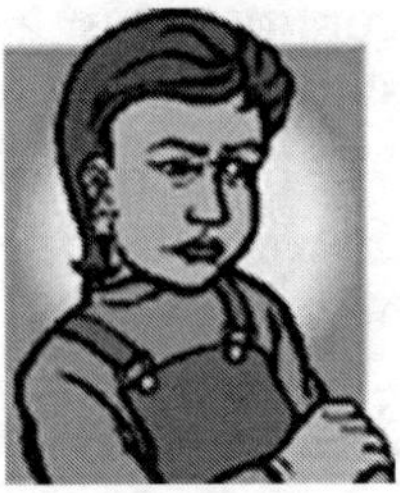

Accept Nothing.....

Change Everything......

and

Nothing Changes

These states are not something achieved, for we have no power to achieve them. They arrive, unannounced, at our door. The m3health Program prepares us for their arrival.

Our role is to make them welcome.

Please take time to review the characteristics of an *Inquiry*.

31
LETTING GO

What a great idea "letting go of the past" is.

Pity it's impossible....

If it weren't, do you think we'd all be hanging onto all those childhood adaptations which just keep coming back, year after year, decade after decade, millennium after millennium, causing us problems. Do you think we'd be contending with the same old problems in our work, our family, and our relationships. And do you think we'd pass on the same old habits to our own children, if we could just drop it! Of course not!

And do you think we'd be suffering from the same old emotional and psychological problems, the same old self-doubts and the same old criticisms of ourselves and others if we could just let go!

And would we be suffering from the same old illnesses?

Not likely....

Letting go is impossible when we attempt it by applying the control we try and exercise over much else in our lives.

It's impossible when we try to *do* it.

Letting go is something that we explore, and which happens to us in the course of the exploration. It's a consequence of being prepared to enter into, and remain within, the Inquiry.

Letting go is something over which we have no control.

If we do have control over it, we aren't letting go.

Remaining within the inquiry which is the m3health Program is the same as allowing life, opening up to life's ups and downs and allowing the excitement of life to infect us.

***We've all been immunised against life,
now's the time to get infected again.***

A breakdown of the term "letting go" suggests that we allow "go" to happen, not make it happen. We allow movement, we become open for movement.... for change..... for evolution. We're not "making go", we're "letting go", or "allowing go".

A better expression than "letting go" might be "exploring becoming available to be let gone of..." Hmmmm.........my editor won't like that one so I'm left with "letting go". Not to worry. If I use the term "let go" you'll know what I mean, as much as language allows one person to communicate with another and as much as accurate communication is actually desirable.

***Perhaps you're better off not knowing
what I really mean, irrelevant as it is to you, or
worse still, limiting of you.***

And the advantage of letting go?

The freeing of the body's healing systems to operate fully.

I've said before that there may be diseases that are so virulent that the human organism can't yet combat them. HIV might be a contemporary example, but even with something as powerful as the HIV virus, there's evidence that some people have successfully fought off the virus using their own immune system.

Letting go is a vital part of letting our illness go, providing the opportunity for it to disappear in a manner similar to that in which it appeared — out of our consciousness and beyond our intention. The m3health Program is a framework for letting go.

By focusing upon the Inquiry we allow the letting go to happen, not make it happen, not force it to happen and not will it to happen.

32
"Ah...Control... How I Love It!"

The problem with it is........the same control we exercise over our lives is busy controlling and restraining our healing mechanisms.

Well.....what to do about that?

Ah now.......there's the "do" word again.

OK......OK......stop bugging me about this.....you know what I mean...how can I contribute to the freeing of my immune response by taking a look at "my control issues"?

Is that better....???

"Yes, you're right......sorry to be so pedantic..."

Let's take a look at one of society's most condemnatory phrases, up there with "anger is dangerous". I'm referring to the ubiquitous.....

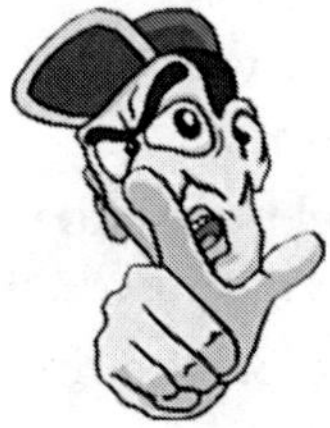

"He's out of control!!"

Now when was the last time you heard that phrase said with a celebratory tone? Either a long time ago or never, I suspect.

Here's a different take on it.

Imagine that "control" is a personal prison keeping its inmate away from the only thing that might heal him....an open communion with his own first nature and a non-separateness from the natural world.

"Control" is his jailer and his prison.

It provides the walls of his defences and threatens him whenever he's tempted to experience life on the outside, where he may achieve freedom from the controls, the known and the expected.

Imagine that "control" is specifically and determinedly keeping you ill?

How does "getting out of control" sound now?

A little better?

Take one little thing.....however minor and non-threatening, but over which you like to exercise control. Think about taking the risk of letting this little thing go and see what happens if you do. Note how it feels.

Can you come up with something?

Here's a few suggestions to get you started......

- Don't ask your wife or husband where she/he's been when she/he comes home at an unexpected time.
- Allow an employee to take a decision on a matter without consulting you.
- Let someone get on with organising an event without you having any input at all.
- See if you can travel by cab to your work without telling the cab driver which route to take or how to drive better.
- Don't interrupt a conversation when you come into a room.

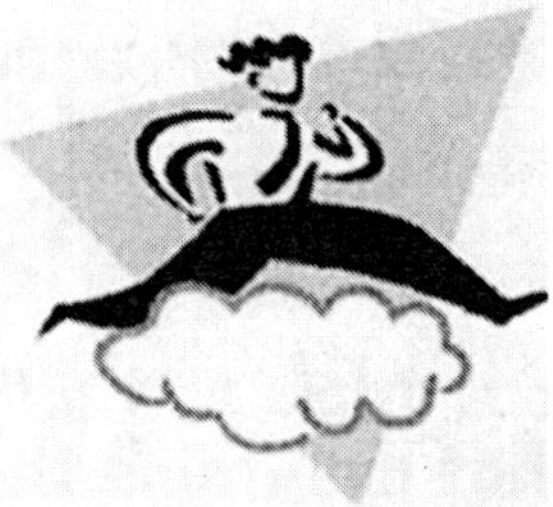

- Let your tennis partner go to the net when he wants to.
- Trust that your child will not spill his drink on the couch.

Have a bit of fun with it.

Before you know it you'll be hanging a sign on your door....

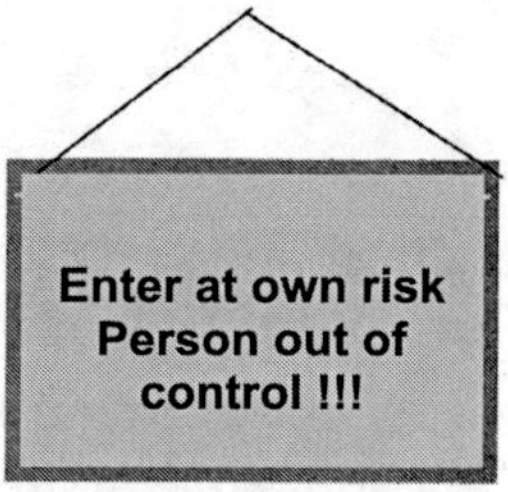

Unless we take the risk of allowing life to heal us, we'll be forever trying to work out how to do it.

It's very difficult for us to divine if either:

- A preferred way exists.
- We're capable of achieving it.

Neither may be correct.

Experiencing the emotions which accompany being out of control may be much more valuable than acquiring "answers" to these questions.

33
Guilt, Fault and Blame

Psstt......Wanna control everyone?

Want to manage a political and legal process that maintains the status quo and alienates well intentioned disrupters?

Ahhh...thank goodness for good old guilt, fault and blame, the trustworthy allies of religion, politics (medical and otherwise) and the law, everywhere.... always.

Many years ago one of our colleagues here at m3health was confronted with a doctor on a talkback radio show. The doctor said that the sort of medicine we were proposing was wrong because it made people feel guilty.

She claimed that people were made to feel guilty because they'd become ill in the first place and then, to make matters worse, they'd failed to recover, a double whammy of guilt. Her view was that most people, if given a choice, would prefer to succumb to their disease, supported by a doctor or loved ones who assured them that the disease was not their fault.

That disease is not the fault of the sufferer is a cornerstone of this book.

However, any resignation which accompanies this sentiment may not be conducive to recovery. Resignation may seem preferable to an often arduous and frightening m3health Inquiry about the nature of illness and our relationship to it. The Inquiry brings the guilt feelings to the surface where, for progress, they must be identified, experienced and brought into the Inquiry process. Better, the doctor believed, to support the patient in suppressing these thoughts and feelings, whatever the medical consequences. She believed that they were not accessible to the sufferer and therefore could play no part in their recovery. Releasing them simply created more suffering.

She was right that many people respond to the m3health Program with feelings of guilt.

We've always devoted a good deal of time in public forums and in private sessions to de-commissioning and then recommissioning the guilt feelings that many people carry for the whole of their lives. This way, feelings of guilt became an asset rather than a liability.

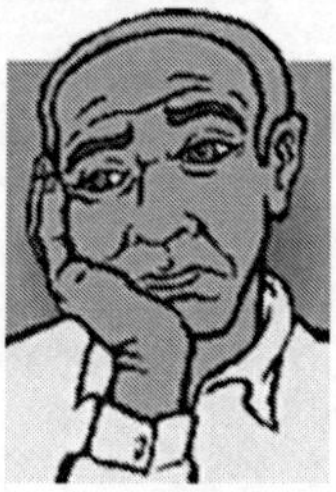

Nothing anyone can say <u>makes</u> us feel guilty....

We're already guilty.

We'll use anything to keep feeling guilty as long as it reinforces our guilt feelings from childhood. We do this to feel the safety of the known. Of course it makes us feel miserable as well.

Fear underlies guilt, fault and blame. Anger directed at oneself might account for guilt..... and anger directed at someone else is a feature of blame. Since we've postulated that fear underlies anger and that the degree to which we find fault with others is the degree to which, deep down, we find fault with ourselves, we can assume that guilt, fault and blame have a common origin within the poor reflection the child makes upon himself given his childhood circumstances. He's loathe to give these up because he's become accustomed to the safety that these beliefs afford, i.e. they've become second nature, and he's mostly unwilling to shed these defences and risk the unknown without them. He'll most likely have attracted a partner equally unwilling to see him move beyond his early childhood guilt, fearing an unwanted development within the partnership if he does. Such an evolution usually means a loss of control of the relationship exercised by his partner. A husband or wife who claims that "I'm miserable and it's your fault"...... is very attractive to a guilty person.

People who play a game of "helpless" attract guilty partners who spend their whole lives trying to make their partner happy.

Here's a summary of m3health's view of guilt.

- If your personality contributed to the development of your own illness it did so for the most honourable of reasons.
- If you continue to feel guilt now over your illness, bring it into your inquiry and it will be one of your most valuable assets.
- If you elect to continue feeling guilty......we continue to honour you.

34

"What should I Do?"

"Should" & "Ought"

"What should I do?" is a very commonly asked question.

Understandable too, as we're afraid of making a mistake and afraid of the consequences for our health if we do. However, the freedom required by our physiology to heal us is not helped by the burden of us being told to do this or do that.

Better to express the fear and anguish of not knowing what to do.

The following expression explains it.

What you should be doing
Is what you are doing.
What you ought to have done
Is what you did.

Going Further

The m3health Program is available

- In this book
- At www.m3health.com

A subscription to the website includes a number of additional features.

1. An online assessment tool, m3checkit.

M3checkit enables you to monitor your journey along the Highway to Health. We all want to know how we're doing when we take on something new and we've been "at it" for a while. Are we making progress? It feels as though something has changed, but has it really?

This is an opportunity to stop driving forward and to reflect on where you've been and consider the progress that you've made. It's time for a breather, time to give yourself some credit for getting where you are, and to put the next stage of your journey into perspective.

M3checkit appears at the end of each chapter of the program and evokes the healing essence from within the participant.

2. An electronic diary, m3diary

M3diary helps to map your progress. The diary contains a section for direct input into the *Personal Report* (see later).

You keep a record of what chapter you found most significant and your impressions of issues which arise in the course of the m3health Program.

Discussions with friends, health attendants or other interested parties can be recorded here, as well as progress noted when re-taking individual chapters. The tool provides a helpful comparison of where you are now, with where you've been, and provides pointers for future explorations.

3. The m3 Personal Report

If you'd like to discuss your personal situation with a convenor from m3health, we'd be happy to assist you. We have conducted health and life issues correspondence with clients for over twenty years, covering a wide range of physical and psychological diseases and personal problems including relationship, business, parenting and sexual problems. Both subscriber and m3health respondent remain anonymous. The subscriber determines the frequency of communication as well as its content.

The Personal Report is deliverable by email only

If you would like to purchase either of these m3 Reports and you don't have your own computer or internet connection you can use an Internet café or perhaps a friend's computer.

FAQ

How soon will I recover?

Everyone differs in his response, but in general you can expect that when you begin to see your disease in a different light your recovery is on the way. The timeframe is not able to be predicted, ranging from immediate to years.

What can I expect?

This is impossible to predict. It depends upon who you are and the nature of your disease. The m3health Program is an exploration. As such you will be discovering the answers to that question yourself, or moving beyond needing to know.

Why should I pay m3health to explore these issues?

Developing and managing the m3health website is a professional undertaking, involving many people. M3health receives no advertising revenue of any kind as we believe it must remain independent to best serve the health interests of its participants. This differentiates it from practically every other health program, health website or health claim. The m3health Program is most effective when used as a companion to your usual therapy, and with the support of your usual medical attendant.

How do I know when my m3health Program is completed?

This is a very interesting question. Many years of experience have shown us that people become fascinated with looking at their lives through new eyes and repeatedly come back to the principles of m3health. Awareness adds up over time. As for the resolution of the symptoms which initiated the m3health Program in the first place, we've noticed that often a third party is required to inform the subscriber that the disease has gone, as the subscriber's focus has moved on from the physical symptoms of the disease. As long as we remain occupied by our disease, we're not yet healed. When we're no longer aware of it, we're healed. This can be a slightly frustrating realisation for those of us concerned with goals and achievements.

What conditions are responsive to the m3health Program?

The m3health Program may be used to address any condition.

It's not helpful to list particular diseases or symptoms because the manifestation of an individual's life journey and the symptoms which accompany it, whatever label they've been assigned, are available to be explored. Long-standing complaints of a serious or life threatening nature are more difficult to access, but on the other hand, there's often more motivation to explore them.

Should I give up my normal medical treatment whilst undertaking the m3health Program?

No.

The m3health Program is an adjunct to medical therapy, and the subscriber is responsible for his ongoing medical treatment whilst undertaking the m3health Program. When the medical condition subsides or disappears, the subscriber should discuss this development with his usual medical attendant.

Can the m3health Program be used to prevent illness?

Yes.

The m3health Program is intended to be used for the recovery from illness and the prevention of its recurrence along with the maintenance of general good health.

Will my discomfort increase whilst I undertake the m3health Program?

Perhaps.

One reason we need assistance in undertaking the m3health Program is that we're afraid to look at matters that might be playing a part in our disease. When we take the risk of looking at our illness differently we may experience a range of feelings such as anger, sadness, fear and joy, as well as some of the bodily discomforts that go with them. The increase in discomfort is temporary. The longer term effects are improved health, less physical discomfort, and peace of mind.

For simplicity m3health uses ″he″ and “she″ interchangeably.

About Us

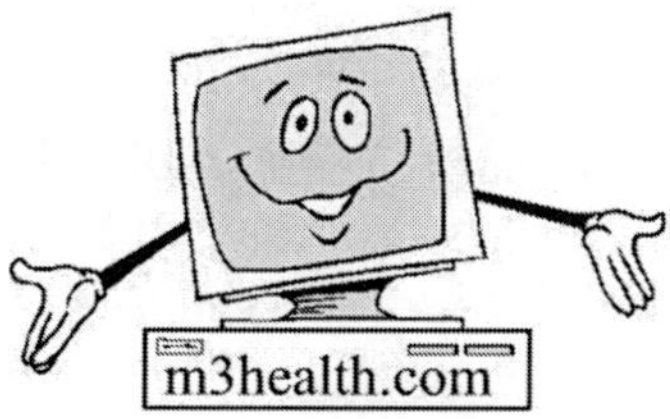

M3health, Health in the Third Millennium, believes that we need new ways of looking at health.

M3health believes that optimal health is achieved by the patient playing his part in both his recovery from disease, and the maintenance of his own health.

Your usual medical attendant completes the team assembled to assist you.

M3health sells no products, potions, drugs, remedies or medicaments. Nor does it advocate any system of medicine, orthodox or alternative. It has no religious affiliations and does not recommend individual practitioners. It receives no advertising revenue from any source. This enables m3health to make available health programs based solely upon the health needs of its subscribers.

M3health focuses on helping people help themselves.

Anonymity for both m3health convenors and m3health participants is maintained for the benefit of both, and for the maintenance of the relationship between participants and their usual health attendants.

For those readers wanting direct personal contact with a convenor of m3health, please visit the website www.m3health.com

The section "Going further" (page 196) in this book describes these options.

To learn more about subscribing, follow the easy instructions on the website by clicking the "Subscription Information" page on the side bar menu on the front page of the website.

You will be given more information to help you and if you elect to subscribe will be taken through a series of simple steps.

Best wishes

M3health